The Sleep Advantage

The Sleep Advantage

OPTIMIZE YOUR NIGHT
TO WIN YOUR DAY

DEVIN BURKE

The Sleep Advantage
Optimize Your Night to Win Your Day

© 2020 Devin Burke

I. Title
The following information is intended as a general reference tool for understanding the underlying principles and practices of the subject matter. The opinions and ideas expressed herein are solely those of the author. This book is not intended to replace recommendations or advice from physicians or other healthcare providers. Instead, it is designed to help you make new decisions about your health to perform at your absolute best.

The strategies outlined in this book may not be suitable for every individual and are not guaranteed or warranted to produce any particular results.

If you are interested in bulk purchases of The Sleep Advantage, we offer an excellent bulk discount. Please email the author at info@devinburke.com.

Editing by Amanda Rogers and Marlene Burke.

Cover photo credit by Kirk Francis.

Printed in the United States of America

ISBN: 978-0-578-75248-8

Interior Design by FormattedBooks.com

To all those who choose to share their gifts to make the world better

Table of Contents

Preface

Could sleep be the key to unlocking how incredible our body and mind are designed to feel?

Is sleep really that important to our health and performance?

When I set out on my journey to discover how to feel my best both physically and mentally over a decade ago, I had no idea that sleep would be such an essential piece of the puzzle. In January 2011, I embarked on a two-and-a-half-month backpacking trip through Europe, which changed my life.

I had just graduated from Florida Atlantic University with a Bachelor of Science in Exercise and Health Promotion with the hope of continuing my education to become a Doctor of Physical Therapy.

At the time, I worked as an exercise tech at a local sports medicine clinic in Boca Raton, FL, while taking the doctoral program prerequisites and prepping for the entry tests.

I was thrilled to be accepted into a Physical Therapy Doctoral Program and decided before jumping back into an intense three year accelerated program, that I should take a vacation. So, I bought a backpack and a one-way ticket to Amsterdam.

During my travels all over Europe, I had time to think about what I wanted and who I wanted to be. After some honest self-reflection and inquiry, I realized that I wasn't that passionate about becoming a Doctor of Physical Therapy, something I had thought I wanted to be since high school.

Shortly after returning from my adventure, while meditating on a beach, I finally decided that I wouldn't pursue something that was out of alignment with my heart's true desire, and I declined my acceptance.

I'll never forget the pit in my stomach after making the phone call to decline my enrollment. Now what? Life always has a way of working itself out. Just a few weeks after making that call, I discovered a holistic health coaching program that was heavily focused on nutrition and life-style management. After speaking with one of their recent graduates and an admissions officer, I immediately enrolled and spent the next year and a half learning how everything we consume - including what we allow into our minds - affects our health and wellbeing.

This program set me on a personal journey to discover how to thrive not just financially, but spiritually and in health and relationships. After attending many personal development seminars, taking courses and workshops, and training with many different mentors, I eventually discovered my purpose *to inspire and lead others to wake up with more peace, power, and presence.*

Over the past decade, I studied and experimented with many different dietary theories, healing modalities, therapies, mindfulness, and meditation techniques. I put my TV behind the couch and began reading hundreds of books on nutritional science, exercise physiology, stress management, psychology, mindfulness, spirituality, and eventually sleep science.

Sleep was the missing link. Like most people who sleep well, I didn't think too much about it. I believed that sleep wasn't that important and that it certainly wasn't a key to accessing deeper levels of awareness, creativity, intelligence, energy, or mental performance. Sleep was just something that happened every night.

It wasn't until a client reached out and asked me if I had ever helped anyone overcome insomnia that my eyes were finally opened to the power and importance of sleep.

The strange thing was that up until this point in my education, I hadn't read or heard that much about sleep. Like any curious student, I bought the top-rated sleep books on Amazon and began reading them.

The more I read, the more fascinated I became. **It turns out that sleep is the single most effective thing we can do to reset our brain, body, and health each day.** I discovered that getting quality sleep is an effortless path to a more productive, energized, and joyful life. Sleep improves every aspect of our lives - our health, relationships, careers, and performance. Sleep is the foundation of energy, and energy is the foundation of life.

Sleep is truly one of the best ways we can spend our time protecting our health and sanity, and accelerating our overall performance.

As I began experimenting with my sleep and felt the effects of improving the quality of my nights significantly improving the quality of my days, I got certified as a Sleep Science Coach. I founded Sleep Science Academy, which helps people who have insomnia and high achievers get and stay asleep using a unique holistic approach based in science.

There are so many factors that affect our health, energy, and performance: our genetics, the type, quality, and amount of food we consume, how we move our bodies, how we manage stress, how we think about ourselves and others, and most importantly, the amount and quality of sleep we get each night.

The truth is that most of us are operating way below our capacity. There is another level for you, and to get there, you'll need to rest. I know that sounds a bit counter-intuitive, but you'll find through reading this book and taking action on the strategies and tools I share in it, how true that statement is.

I've also discovered that consistently feeling our very best comes down to managing with intention three areas - our energy, focus, and time. When we are well slept, we have more power, improved concentration, and make better decisions to spend our time doing more of what matters and less of what doesn't.

When most people think of feeling, looking, and performing at their best, they think of having lots of energy, not the artificial, nervous, coffee-kind of energy, but calm, directed, focused energy, or what I call 'sustained energy.' You may have experienced this type of energy while immersed in a passion project or while on vacation after a great night's sleep. Maybe you woke up feeling physically recharged, mentally clear, and emotionally connected.

Before we dive into all the ways to create more peace, power, and presence by improving your sleep, let's clarify why you decided to read this book. Maybe your goal is to be able to fall asleep faster, rest deeper, wake up with more energy, or feel more confidence and joy. Or perhaps you picked up this book because you're looking to have consistent sustained focus to accomplish more in less time.

When you get great sleep, you gain an edge because great sleep is a superpower. So let's get clear now about why finding your energy edge - how much peace, power, and presence you bring to your day - is important now?

Answer the following questions:

- What does *your best* look like and feel like? What are three words to describe this version of yourself?
- Why is improving your sleep and energy important now?
- In the past three months, how has your physical, mental, and emotional energy felt? Why do you think that is so?

Awareness is the first step to change. I hope by now it's clear that this isn't just a book about sleep. It's a road map to generating effortless energy to live more through unlocking the power of sleep.

Uncovering what the best version of you would look and feel like is the first step toward creating him or her. Connecting to a strong 'why' is essential to keeping you emotionally connected and taking intelligent action toward your vision. Identifying what has been getting in your way will help you get clear on what must change.

Everything we do requires energy, and *sleep* **is the foundation of health and vitality.** Here are a few more questions to help you get even more clear:

- What could you do with more energy?
- What will experiencing increased clarity and energy create in your life?
- What are you *willing to do* to generate more energy now?
- What are you *willing to no longer do* to generate more energy now?
- How much time do you spend daily doing things that distract you from restful sleep (e.g., TV, social media, texting, web surfing, etc.)?
- What is the root of these distractions? Stress? Overwhelm? Fear? Disorganization? Lack of discipline?

I've never met anyone (yet) that has shared with me that they wanted to feel low energy, depressed, and unfulfilled. However, so many people today are silently suffering from one or all of these low-energy states because of their unexamined thoughts, beliefs, choices, and habits.

We often know what we could or should be doing, but don't do what we know. This is usually because we haven't taken the time to create a compelling enough vision for our health and life, or if we have, we've lost sight of it. What is your vision for your health and life? Do you have one? If not, stop reading and start getting clear on this now.

Who Is This Book For?

Here are a few questions to help you figure out if this book is right for you:

- Do you want to be able to fall asleep faster, rest deeper, and wake refreshed?
- Do you have low energy during the day or desire more energy?
- Do you find (or do others find) that you're moody or anxious?
- Do you experience cravings for sugar and caffeine?
- Are you struggling with losing weight?
- Have you recently gained weight?
- Do you find that you regularly forget things and desire a sharper mind?
- Is your sex drive or libido low?
- Do you find that small things can cause you to overreact?
- Do you want to tap into a higher level of performance?
- Do you desire a deeper level of connection with friends and family?

If you even checked one of these boxes, then this book is for you. **This book is for those seeking to live a life full of energy, purpose, and pas-**

sion. It's for all those ready to make a change and committed to creating a new standard for their health and life. I hope that's you. And if it is, I'm so glad you decided to pick up this book.

A note on insomnia:

While this book can be helpful for just about everyone, it does not explicitly address the disorder of insomnia. What is insomnia? Insomnia is a sleep disorder where you have trouble falling (onset insomnia) or staying asleep (maintenance insomnia).

Insomnia can be short-term (acute) or can last a long time (chronic). It can also come and go. Acute insomnia lasts from one night to a few weeks. Insomnia is considered 'chronic' when it happens at least three nights a week for three months or more.

About 40 million Americans suffer from some type of insomnia every night. If you have insomnia, please visit **www.SleepScienceAcademy. com** to learn more about how we can support you. We offer programs using a unique holistic approach based on science that has helped hundreds of clients get and stay asleep all night long. Our mission is to give people the tools and support they need to stop suffering and start sleeping as soon as possible. We help our clients get and stay asleep each night, even if they've "tried everything" and have been struggling for years.

Unfortunately, most insomnia 'solutions' available today are simply not sustainable or even effective because they don't address the root causes of insomnia, which in most cases are stress and anxiety related. The most popular mainstream 'treatment' for insomnia is taking sleeping pills, which have dangerous side effects, including increased risk of cancer.

Avoiding the Danger Zone

A healthy person has a thousand desires; a sick person has one. —Indian Proverb

Most of the world, and especially in America, people live in what I call the *danger zone*. The danger zone is living in the state of not being healthy, but not being unhealthy enough to do anything about it.

Sadly, we usually wait to make a much needed and necessary lifestyle change until it's too painful not to. We all too often ignore the signs and symptoms of failing health until something drastic happens, forcing us to change.

I found that most people don't realize how unhealthy they are until they begin to become healthier, and only then realize what they were missing. The reality is that **most people put their health on the back burner until it becomes too painful not to do something about it. This must change.** Please choose to learn from others' mistakes and not let this happen to you! Unfortunately, we typically don't know how amazing we can feel because we're not aware of how bad we currently feel (even if we think we currently feel pretty good). We have become accustomed to poor sleep, impaired health, limited performance, and low energy levels. In other words, exhaustion and semi-poor health become our accepted norm. Although not getting fantastic sleep, feeling low energy, craving sugar, carrying around a few extra pounds, and having brain fog may be the norm, it's far from normal.

Jake was one of the top financial planners for a top financial institution. He was a high performer who excelled at whatever he set his mind to, especially when managing and growing his financial service business. As he pushed his business forward, making more and more money, he ignored the warning signs that his body was giving him to slow down and make changes in his health and life.

He was burning the midnight oil and only sleeping four to five hours a night, and this went on for years. His diet was good but not great, and he did exercise, although he mentioned only as much as his "schedule would allow," and shared with me that he continually sacrificed his sleep for work.

Jake is a perfect example of someone living in the 'danger zone,' and he eventually paid the price. Although he had become financially successful, he went bankrupt in his health and relationships. After a stressful divorce, he was diagnosed with *chronic fatigue syndrome* and *burnout syndrome* (Recognized by the World Health Organization in 2019). When his marriage ended, he lost half his net worth from the divorce and then spent the next seven years and over a half a million dollars trying to reclaim his health. No matter what Jake tried, he still felt tired, fatigued, frustrated, and anxious. It took him many years of pain and suffering and hundreds of thousands of dollars in consulting with some of the world's top doctors and visiting multiple healing institutes around the world to finally figure out how to reclaim his health. He discovered that sleep was a massive foundational key to his healing. Through making his sleep and health his number one priority, he eventually reclaimed his energy edge, and in the process, reconnected to his purpose.

When we are in a low energetic state physically, mentally, or emotionally, we can't bring the best of who we are to our families, friends, businesses, communities, churches, or missions. *Living with purpose* **takes energy, and you can't give that which you don't have. When you take care of your health by prioritizing sleep, you can create the energy necessary to make your greatest impact and enjoy life more fully.** You're able to tap into the best parts of who we are and make your greatest contribution to your family, community, company, and the world.

There is a reason they say on an airplane to put your oxygen mask on first before assisting others, because how are you going to help anyone else if you're unconscious? If your tired, stressed, frustrated, and overwhelmed, how will you give your full presence to your spouse, kids, or at the big meeting? How will you create the energy to do the things you love with the people you love? How can you give them the greatest gift, the gift they deserve, your full presence?

The answer to these questions is most likely no, or at least not at the level you're capable of. One of the biggest mistakes I see in seeking increased health, energy, and performance is trying to tackle too many health pillars at once. It's essential to focus on the health pillar that will make the most significant impact first and generate the most momentum. **If you're currently sacrificing your sleep or not actively improving your sleep quality, *sleep* is that pillar for you.**

Every day, we get the chance to make new choices. We are not bound to old conditions, old patterns, or old ways of thinking, being, or acting, yet we often act as if we are. We are creatures of habit and live into our patterns of the past unless we decide and commit to something new. If we all know that eating healthy, drinking water, managing our stress, moving our bodies, and getting quality sleep is essential to our health, why is it so challenging to maintain these common-sense and straightforward health practices?

The answer is simple: we get in our way. We overanalyze things, which leads to procrastination; then, we make excuses and, even worse, believe them.

> *"There's not enough time."*
> *"I'm just too busy right now."*
> *"It costs too much."*
> *"I'll do it tomorrow, next week, month, year."*

It's time to get out of our way to generate the energy that will help us live with more peace, power, and presence. Life is happening now. If you're looking for a sign to make a massive shift and change your health, life, and performance, this is it!

It's essential to continue to be curious, experiment, test, and be open to new ideas and possibilities to live and feel better. It's often when we question conventional thinking that real breakthroughs and true discoveries happen, even during sleep.

PART 1

Sleep: The Missing Link

Introduction

Sleep is one of those things that we all know we need more of, yet somehow, it seems to get sacrificed. Seventy million Americans currently suffer from some type of sleep disorder, and it appears that we are so tired during work hours that we often become unfulfilled in our jobs and relationships; when, if we just got a bit more shut-eye, things could be so different.

When we don't get enough sleep, we tend to be less productive, moody, forgetful, and crave sugar or fat while having a significant decrease in willpower to resist the sugar and fatty foods. Can you relate?

To make things worse, in today's fast-paced world, there seems to be a badge of honor about how little one can sleep and still function despite the common knowledge that getting regular, consistent sleep is the foundation for a healthy body and life.

"I don't need to sleep."
"I do fine with a few hours of sleep."
"Sleep is a waste of time."
"I'll sleep when I'm dead."
"The early bird gets the worm."
"You snooze, you lose."

How many times have you heard something like this? Or worse, said it yourself? The truth is when you snooze, you actually win, and science now proves it. Yes, we can get by in the short term with a little less sleep, but eventually, it catches up with us, and who wants to just get by anyway? **We get this one precious life, and *just getting by* is not fully tapping into our human potential. Each of us is here to thrive, not just survive!** *Just getting by* often means not contributing our best or often not getting the job done at all.

Tom was a 47-year-old busy executive working for a large corporation. Like many of his high-performing colleagues, Tom had the illusion that sleep was for the lazy and that it was a weak habit of low performers. It was something that maybe others needed, but he didn't have the time for and could do without. As a result of this belief, Tom only slept between 4-5 hours per night, which went on for years.

He didn't realize time spent sleeping is the most critical time for our brain to recover, repair, and reboot. After years of sacrificing his sleep and getting poor quality sleep, he eventually began to feel the result of his decision to sacrifice it. Tom shared with me that he was becoming more forgetful, less focused, and that his sex drive went through the floor; and he felt he was losing his edge, and to be honest, he was. He thought, "well, this must be because I'm getting old."

Over several years, he had put on ten extra pounds of fat around his midsection, and he couldn't seem to lose it no matter what he ate or how much he exercised. He began to rely on coffee and stimulants to get through the day and then resorted to alcohol to calm his nerves at night.

He knew something had to change, but he didn't know where to start. He was becoming more concerned about his performance at work, which caused him to lose even more sleep, resulting in waking up feeling even more stressed, tired, irritable, and fatigued. Eventually, his worst nightmare came true: Tom lost his energy edge, and it cost him his job.

Why am I sharing this story with you? Well, I don't want you to be a 'Tom.' Don't wait until it costs you your job, relationship, or health to make a change in getting the rest your body and brain so desperately need.

To experience how good our bodies and minds are designed to feel, while enjoying the process *versus* suffering through it, we need recovery time and quality sleep. Simply put, when we don't get enough quality sleep, our physical and mental performance *drastically* suffer. There is no doubt: we MUST prioritize and protect our sleep if we wish to experience sustained performance and optimal health.

The scary fact is that most people think that getting sick a few times a year, carrying an extra five to ten pounds around their waist, and tossing and turning all night is normal. Most people believe that waking up feeling tired, sluggish, and having to rely on coffee or other stimulants to get them through their day is also normal. These are all signs that your body is begging for help.

> *We now see sleep as the preeminent force in this health trinity. The physical and mental impairments caused by one night of bad sleep dwarf those caused by an equivalent absence of food or exercise.* —Matthew Walker, *Why We Sleep*

Let me be clear from the start, this book isn't the transformation – it's the map and plan. That being said, I believe in keeping things simple. I believe it's possible to do more with less. In a world obsessed with more, I have found that it's often **the simple choices and changes when done with great consistency, that make the most significant impact.** You can take your sleep and health to the next level by using the simple strategies covered in this book, but it starts with a 100% commitment. Are you committed?

Sleep Science 101

Many people mistakenly believe that sleep is a waste of time because they are ignorant (like I once was) of all the magic that happens when we are asleep. During sleep, our bodies' and brains' waste removal teams visit us and clean up all the day's cellular waste.

Not to get too much in the weeds here, but each night (depending on how long we sleep), we go through several sleep cycles, usually between four to six times per night. Within these sleep cycles, we go through five sleep stages broken into two different categories: REM sleep (dream sleep) and non-REM (NREM) sleep.

Stages of sleep

1. NREM
   a) Stage 1 - Period between wakefulness and sleep. Conscious awareness begins to fade.
   b) Stage 2 - Heart rate slows, and blood pressure drops.
   c) Stage 3-4 (deep sleep) - Hormones are released, and the body removes cellular waste.

2. REM - Increased heart rate, the body is immobilized, and dreams occur.

About every 90-110 minutes, we cycle through these sleep stages with NREM sleep ratio to REM sleep dramatically changing across the night, creating our unique nightly sleep architecture. NREM deep sleep mostly occurs in the first quarter of the night, especially between the hours of 10-12 pm. This type of high-quality sleep boosts our immune system, balances hormones, increases metabolism, and restores physical energy. Deep sleep is vitally important to body and brain recovery. REM sleep usually happens in the middle to the fourth quarter of the night. Our body and brain seem to desire most of their REM sleep in the last part of the night, so not getting enough sleep either because of going to bed too late or waking up too early affects these critical sleep stages.

The 4 Stages of Sleep

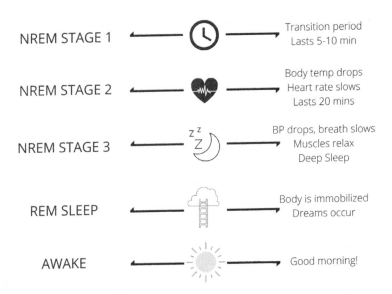

NREM STAGE 1	Transition period Lasts 5-10 min
NREM STAGE 2	Body temp drops Heart rate slows Lasts 20 mins
NREM STAGE 3	BP drops, breath slows Muscles relax Deep Sleep
REM SLEEP	Body is immobilized Dreams occur
AWAKE	Good morning!

Sleep - The Great Performance Enhancer

Sleep enriches a wide range of functions, including our ability to learn, remember, make logical decisions, and maintain stable emotions. It is the single most effective thing we can do each day to reset our brains, bodies, and health.

A lack of sleep creates an accumulation of the sleep chemical *adenosine*. Adenosine is what accumulates in our brains through the day to develop sleep pressure - the body's desire or hunger for sleep. When we don't get enough sleep (kind of like an outstanding debt), adenosine carries over into the next day. It will continue to accumulate with each passing day that we don't get enough sleep, eventually leading to mental and physical burnout. In sleep science, we call this *sleep debt,* and it's a debt that can't be repaid.

It's not enough to just get a certain amount of sleep each night, **we must strive to put in place habits that will support higher quality restorative sleep. It's this kind of sleep quality that especially helps us win our days.**

In our fast-paced, high-tech world, it's no surprise that most of us have trouble falling asleep or staying asleep each night. It's estimated that more than 40% of Americans get less than the recommended *minimum* of seven hours of sleep per night. Not getting enough sleep affects our mental acuity, clarity, and physical energy.

I often hear, "I just can't shut my mind down at night," or "I wake up several times during the night," from clients who are incredibly high-achieving individuals.

Learning new habits and strategies to *switch off* is essential to experiencing sustainable, high-quality sleep each night and high performance during the day. I'll share with you how to retrain your mind to *switch off* in the chapters to come.

The Lure Not to Sleep

With the wonderful invention of electricity, the light bulb, devices like smartphones and iPads, and of course, Netflix and Amazon Prime, the lure of 24-hour-a-day fun or work (knowing somewhere, in some time zone, someone else is working while you indulge in sleep)and the pull to neglect sleep has never been stronger.

In the 21st century, technology is one of the biggest challenges to practicing intelligent self-care and getting seven to eight hours of high-quality sleep. We are addicted to our devices, and sadly these addictions are costing us much more than our precious time and attention. They are costing us our health!

Our attention is being monetized and monopolized, and we are paying the price. For better or worse, technology and social media have massively changed society. They're affecting how we connect and relate, and they are 100% getting in the way of our sleep!

Unfortunately, for most people, sleep is also seen as a weakness to be conquered. This is no surprise since, as a society, we are programmed to think that adequate sleep is a weak habit of low performers. Sleeping is seen as lazy…it's primarily seen as a waste of time.

In today's society, there is a massive disconnect between sleep and its critical function to our health and performance. Causes of sleep deprivation can range from a wide variety of conditions depending on different life circumstances. Some of these include prioritizing work or entertainment over sleep, having a baby, your unique chronobiology, current health history, stressful events like losing a job or going through a divorce, and stress management.

However, for most people, **stress is the number one cause of a lack of sleep**, so we will be exploring the connection between sleep and stress and how to transform stress in the chapters to come in much greater detail.

Why Sleep Is Essential

Most people can agree that sleep is essential, but many don't realize just how critical sleep is for our overall mental and emotional health. Sleep is like taking your car to the garage after a long trip for a comprehensive tune-up and replacement of worn-out parts each night.

Anyone who has experienced a workday following little to no sleep feels the dramatic decrease in focus and clarity in virtually all tasks. But why does our body encourage us to sleep in the first place?

During REM sleep, most brain activity is quite similar to a state of someone while awake. Understanding why we sleep at all has long been a point of scientific contention, with some theories focusing on memory consolidation and others pointing to cognitive processing and recovery. But the one thing that all science does agree on is that sleep is critical.

A lifestyle that doesn't account for adequate sleep (seven to nine hours for most people) can result in severe cognitive impairments and risks. This is because not getting enough sleep impairs the prefrontal cortex, which helps us problem-solve, reason, organize, plan, and execute those plans. It's this part of the brain that helps us make quality decisions and get things done, and **very often, the quality of our lives comes down to the quality of our decisions.**

When we are sleep-deprived, we experience 'cognitive fatigue.' It's this type of mental fatigue that leads to reduced alertness and reaction time and impaired decision-making. This is why we make big mistakes when we are sleep deprived. Sleep deprivation is thought to have played a role in some of the most devastating mistakes in history. The Space Shuttle Challenger explosion, which killed seven crew members, the Exxon Valdez oil spill, which caused the deaths of hundreds of thousands of birds and sea creatures, and the Three Mile Island Nuclear Plant disaster have all been linked to sleep deprivation.

Much like a computer during the night, sleep provides the opportunity for our brains to reboot. This reboot allows us to process higher-level cognitive tasks such as learning, decision-making, and reasoning throughout our day.

Getting enough sleep helps us effectively solve problems while supporting our ability to come up with innovative and creative ideas.

Other research has established that creative thinking occurs during dream sleep, enhancing the integration of unassociated information, and promoting innovative solutions. For example, Paul McCartney came up with the lyrics for the song *Yesterday* in a dream; Dmitri Mendeleev got the idea of the periodic table from a dream; Mary Shelley dreamed the idea for the book *Frankenstein*, and Elias Howe got the idea to finish the invention of the sewing machine in a dream. **Dreaming creates an opportunity for innovation and breakthroughs to take place during the night.**

Getting enough quality sleep also acts as an emotional first aid. When we get the sleep we need, our brains are better able to process emotions and emotional events. Getting enough sleep also allows us to better express our feelings. When **we sleep well, we are better partners, parents, friends, and family members.**

Another client I helped was Susan, a 38-year-old wife and mother of three. She was always so busy trying to juggle running an online business, raising her kids, and managing a household while her husband was gone all day at work. Susan felt that there were never enough hours in the day to complete her tasks, let alone sleep. Susan was what I call a 'get-it-all-done girl.' She would put everyone else's needs before her own, and it eventually caught up with her. When I asked her, Susan couldn't remember the last time she had a good night's rest. She felt tired, irritable, and on edge all the time, and she was so ready for a change!

Susan's lack of sleep caused her to be short with her husband and kids, leaving her feeling guilty for being so moody with those she cared about most. Susan admitted she had lost her energy edge, and her family was paying the price.

After I explained to Susan in one of my seminars that sleep was the key to getting her energy edge back and that without energy, she wouldn't be able to bring her best self to her family, she decided to make her sleep and health her top priority. Within a few weeks of changing her focus to intelligent self-care, Susan's brain fog lifted, her youthful energy returned, her skin looked radiant, and her business began to take off. Susan slept her way back to finding her energy edge.

How Sleep Boosts Our Immune System

One of the most significant benefits of getting great sleep is how it increases longevity and our immune system's health. Quality sleep slows down the aging process by keeping our telomeres healthy. Telomeres are the caps at the end of chromosomes that protect our cells and genes. As we age, they naturally begin to shorten, but studies show that quality sleep slows this shortening effect keeping those caps long and us looking and feeling young.

Many studies have proven the immune-boosting effects of quality sleep, but how does sleep strengthen our immune system exactly?

When we get seven to nine hours a night of quality sleep, our body makes cells called cytokines. Cytokines are a type of protein that targets infection and inflammation, thus activating our immune system. Cytokines are both produced and released during sleep.

A 2019 study published in the Journal of Experimental Medicine found that quality sleep also improves T cells. T cells are the cells that fight viruses such as the flu, herpes, and even cancerous cells. They play an especially important role in the body's immune system. The study found a new way that sleep assists the immune system.

The researchers found that quality sleep promotes the stickiness of a class of adhesion molecules called integrins. This stickiness is vital because for T cells to kill infected, diseased cells such as cancer cells, they need to get in direct contact with them, and the integrin stickiness promotes this contact.

The researchers compared T cells from healthy volunteers who either slept or stayed awake all night. The study found that participants who slept had T cells showing higher levels of integrin activation than in the T cells of those who were awake all night. The findings indicate that sleep has the potential to enhance T cell functioning.

For people who get inadequate sleep, stress hormones stay high and may inhibit T cells' ability to function as effectively. Interestingly, it's been found that chronic sleep loss even makes the flu vaccine less effective by hindering the body's ability to fight off the virus. This is another excellent reason to protect and prioritize sleep!

Quality sleep has been found to:

1. Activate the release of human growth hormone (HGH), an essential player in cellular regeneration and healthy aging.
2. Enhance memory function and creative problem-solving skills the next day.
3. Support athletic performance, including speed, agility, and overall energy.
4. Boost the immune system, leaving us less vulnerable to illness.
5. Help us be more resilient to daily stress.
6. Support a positive mood and outlook on life.
7. Accelerate fat loss.
8. Help speed up recovery from physical activities.

Better quality sleep will help you:

- Be a higher-performing, more creative entrepreneur.
- Become a more patient, attentive, and present spouse or partner.
- Be a more compassionate, kind, and caring parent.
- Perform better sexually.
- Enjoy life more, which in turn makes you and everyone around you happier.

Sleep Experiment

Take action: Think of a few reasons why making sleep a priority is essential for you now. Choose something that resonates with you. Then, set the alarm on your phone for an hour before you plan to go to bed. Just like we set alarms to wake us up in the morning, we must start setting alarms to get to bed at night. This 'sleep alarm' will help remind you of all your reasons for why getting a good night's sleep is essential and help you jumpstart your new sleep bedtime ritual, which we'll discuss in later chapters in more detail.

Sleep - The Ultimate Fat Burner

Can you guess where most of your fat-burning takes place? Hint: it's not at the gym. It's during stage 4 delta sleep! Sleep is not the only factor in sustaining weight loss, but it's a super important key that is often overlooked.

A study conducted at the University of Chicago put participants on a calorie-restricted diet for eight weeks. One group slept 5.5 hours a night, and the comparison group slept 8.5 hours a night. The group that slept for at least 8 hours lost 55% more body fat, with all other factors remaining constant, than the group that had restricted sleep.

Here is why sleep is the ultimate fat burner: A lack of sleep...

1. Decreases your willpower, leading to poor nutritional choices.
2. Causes your body to hold onto fat, hampering your metabolism and contributing to weight gain.
3. Lowers your energy to fuel workouts and recover from them.

Getting inadequate sleep sets your brain up to make bad decisions. As you know, it affects the brain's frontal lobe, the control center of decision-making and impulse control. So, while you may be able to control comfort food cravings when you're well-rested, it's much harder when you're overtired.

A study in the American Journal of Clinical Nutrition found that when people were starved of sleep, late-night snacking increased and they were more likely to choose high-carb snacks. A second study titled, "Sleep and Obesity," found that sleeping too little also prompts people to eat larger portions of food, thus increasing caloric intake and weight gain. And in a review of 18 studies, researchers found that a lack of sleep led to increased cravings for foods specifically high in carbohydrates.

This is because too little sleep triggers an increase in the stress hormone cortisol. Cortisol signals your body to conserve energy to fuel your waking hours and causes your body to hang on to fat. And if that wasn't enough, researchers from the University of Chicago found that sleep deprivation makes us 'metabolically groggy.' They found that within just four days of insufficient sleep, our body's ability to effectively use insulin (the master storage hormone) becomes completely disrupted. Insulin sensitivity, the researchers found, dropped by more than 30%! When your body becomes insulin-resistant, your body has trouble processing fats from your bloodstream, so it ends up storing them as fat.

Hunger is controlled by two hormones: leptin and ghrelin. Leptin is a hormone that makes you feel full. Ghrelin is the hormone that makes you feel hungry. Research published in the Journal of Clinical Endocrinology and Metabolism found that sleeping less than six hours triggers the area of your brain that increases your need for food while also depressing leptin and stimulating ghrelin.

In other words, you crave sugar and fat like crazy, and still feel hungry even after eating! In a nutshell, not getting enough sleep makes us always hungry, eat bigger portions, and desire all the foods that contribute to weight gain while destroying our willpower to stop eating them.

Poor Sleep Sabotages Muscle

Muscle is the enemy of fat—poor sleep is the enemy of muscle. Scientists from Brazil found that sleep debt decreases protein synthesis (your body's ability to make muscle), causes muscle loss, and can lead to a higher incidence of injuries.

A lack of sleep also makes it harder for your body to recover from exercise by slowing down the production of the Human Growth Hormone (HGH)—the anti-aging and fat-burning hormone released in delta slow-wave sleep. As I mentioned previously, a poor night of rest increases the stress hormone cortisol, which slows down the production of HGH.

That means that the already reduced production of growth hormone due to lack of slow-wave sleep is further reduced by more cortisol in your system. When you're suffering from sleep debt, everything you do feels more challenging, especially your workouts because a lack of sleep increases your perception of pain by 15%.

Sleep and Hormones

Hormones are the master information communicators in the body. They control much of what goes on in our bodies and are the keys to optimal sleep, health, and energy. Almost everything that happens in the body can be traced back to hormones. Hormones control our blood sugar levels and affect our heart rate, blood pressure, respiratory rate, and metabolism, as well as our emotional health, ability to focus, sex drive, and reproduction.

The effect of hormones on sleep and sleep on hormones is drastic. For example, studies have shown that poor sleep effectively *ages* a man by 10-15 years in terms of testosterone virility. It was also found that men who have poor quality sleep have 29% lower sperm count, an increase in sperm deformities, and even have significantly smaller testicles than those who sleep well. Yikes! Also, routinely sleeping less than six hours a night resulted in a 20% drop in follicular releasing hormone in women, which is necessary for conception.

Physiologically, sleep occurs when the synchronization and balance of essential hormones are produced and released in our bodies at the right times. Each of the hormones below plays a vital role in improving sleep quality. The way to balance these hormones is to follow the practices laid out for you in this book. The more you prioritize sleep and practice good sleep hygiene and healthy lifestyle habits, the quicker these hormones will be optimized.

Cortisol is often associated with stress and given a bad reputation, but the truth is that cortisol isn't the enemy. We need it, especially after exercise or during stressful situations. Cortisol manages our bodies' daily rhythms. The key to optimizing cortisol is making sure it's released at the right times and in the correct amounts. When your body is in sync with its natural rhythms and you're practicing stress mastery, your cortisol levels should be highest around 6 am and then drop to their lowest levels around 10 pm. Research shows that after several nights of sleep deprivation, cortisol can become elevated at night and contribute to restless sleep.

Human growth hormone (HGH) is an incredible longevity hormone that is released the most during the first half of our sleep in the delta sleep or NREM stage 3. **Research shows that as much as 75% of the human growth hormone is released during sleep.** Slow-wave delta sleep is when we achieve our deepest sleep and when our bodies restore the most. HGH aids in building lean muscle, burns fat, protects our muscles from breaking down, and gives us energy.

Melatonin, also known as the sleep hormone, signals the body that it's time for sleep. It's produced by the pineal gland in the brain and is triggered by darkness and suppressed by exposure to natural and artificial light. We will explore the effects of lighting and sleep in the chapters to come.

Serotonin is a neurotransmitter that plays a crucial role in regulating mood and sleep-wake cycles. Healthy levels of serotonin contribute to a positive mood and outlook and also promote restful sleep. One critical way that serotonin affects sleep is through its relationship with the sleep hormone, melatonin. Melatonin is made from serotonin in the presence of darkness.

Norepinephrine is involved in the synthesis of melatonin and plays a crucial part in balancing the body's overall stress response. Norepinephrine is secreted during REM sleep stages.

Another perfect example of how hormones affect sleep quality is how they affect sleep in peri and postmenopausal women. Menopause is driven by the decline in the production of the hormones estrogen, progesterone, and testosterone. The changing and decreasing levels of these hormones cause many menopausal symptoms, including hot flashes -- body temperature rises usually accompanied by an awakening. Women report the most sleeping problems during this time of life, and generally, postmenopausal women are less satisfied with their sleep. As many as 61% report insomnia symptoms. According to the 2017 Center for Disease Control and Prevention survey, sleep problems tend to increase significantly during perimenopause.

- More than half of perimenopausal women—56%—sleep less than seven hours a night, on average.
- Nearly one-quarter—24.8%—of perimenopausal women say they have trouble falling asleep four or more times a week.
- Even more common than trouble falling asleep is difficulty staying asleep. Among women in perimenopause, 30.8% say they have difficulty staying asleep at least four nights a week.
- Half of perimenopausal women—49.9%—wake in the morning feeling tired, rather than feeling rested four or more days in a week.[1]

What these statistics show clearly is how much hormones truly do affect our sleep. The good news is by focusing on more and better sleep, we can help our bodies stay hormonally balanced throughout life.

---

[1]   To learn more and get support around sleep and menopause visit www.SleepScienceAcademy.com

PART 2

Mastering Sleep

Your Sleep Is Unique to You

Chronobiology is the study of circadian rhythm and its effect on human health and wellness. Circadian rhythm is your biological clock or schedule, which includes the ebb and flow of hormones, enzymes, and body temperature among many other bodily functions.

Each of us has a master biological (bio) clock synchronizing our body and brain activities over the course of 24 hours. Yet, interestingly, researchers have found that we have different 'chronotypes' or biological clock variances, which are unique to us based on our genetics. For instance, you probably have heard of the terms 'night owl' and 'morning lark.' These are the most popular names for chronotype classifications for evening types and morning types.

According to Dr. Michael Breus, Ph.D., *"Our sleep drive is genetic, and it determines how much sleep we need and the depth of sleep."* He states that our chronotype is determined specifically by the PER3 gene. If you have a long PER3 gene, you need at least seven hours of sleep to function and tend to be an early riser. If you have a short PER3 gene, you can get by on less sleep and tend to be a late riser. Based on his research, he has identified four different chronotypes and has named them according to mammals in the wild that accurately represent the four unique bio clocks categories. Based on his findings, each type of chronotype has unique 'chrono rhythms' or daily schedules that, when followed, greatly benefit a person's sleep, health, and well-being.

Below are the four different chronotypes he has defined:

1. Dolphins - usually insomniacs, neurotic light sleepers with low sleep drive.
2. Lions - morning type, driven optimist with medium sleep drive.
3. Bears - good sleepers with high sleep drive.
4. Wolves - night oriented, creative extroverts with medium sleep drive.

In his best-selling book, *The Power of When*, Dr. Breus shares how to maximize your life based on your unique chronobiology. Based on the understanding of our biology and unique circadian rhythm, we can learn when to get the most out of ourselves. In his fascinating book, he touches on the best times to exercise, eat, have sex, do creative work, and of course, go to sleep and wake up.[2]

---

[2] To learn more about chronobiology and to discover what type you are visit www. PowerofWhenQuiz.com

We Manage What We Measure

We are living in a fantastic time in history, the age of the 'quantified self.'

Although most technology is getting in the way of a great night's sleep, some technology is helping us improve it. A few years ago, we didn't have the tech to measure and track our sleep accurately. You'd have to spend the entire night in a sleep lab to see what was going on with your sleep.

But with today's technological advancements in wearable devices, we can now accurately measure relevant sleep data like sleep stages, body temperature, sleep latency, and sleep efficiency. These devices can even measure heart rate variability (the time between each heartbeat) and tell us how well our bodies are recovering.

What's measured gets managed. Having access to this type of sleep data at our fingertips allows us to make new educated decisions and directly see the effect of those decisions on our sleep. We can see how drinking a big glass of wine before bed disrupts REM sleep and how dropping the temperature of our bedroom helps support deep sleep. With this type of daily feedback, we can learn how to improve our sleep and better understand our bodies to reach our health goals even faster. This type of feedback allows us to optimize the most critical aspects of our well-being and motivates us to continue to make decisions that support our sleep and health rather than detract from them.

The device I use and recommend to all my clients is called the Oura Ring. I found this stylish ring to be one of the most accurate wearable sleep-tracking device on the market today. As you read this book, I highly recommend investing in this cutting-edge wearable and utilizing it as you try out the suggested sleep experiments.

Important note: A new term for those obsessed with sleep tracking is called orthosomnia—a "perfectionist's quest to achieve perfect sleep." If tracking your sleep is doing more harm than good, then stop tracking it and seek support at www.SleepScienceAcademy.com.

The Pyramids of Health and Sleep

To experience how good our body and mind are designed to feel, we must take a holistic and systematic approach to health and well being. Our bodies are an amazing interconnected series of systems that all support and work together to sustain life.

Energy is everything. It controls how we think, feel, and more times than not, it controls what we do, which determines our results. Simply put, **the better we feel, the better we perform.** Without energy, nothing gets accomplished. Without energy, we cannot fulfill our purpose to expand, grow, and contribute. It's a natural law that nothing gets accomplished without the proper transference of energy.

The foundation of energy is sleep. We can last a few minutes without air, a few days without water, about a week without sleep, about a month without food, and a few years without exercise before our bodies completely shut down. Nature has shown us the priority order to sustain life is air, water, sleep, food, then exercise.

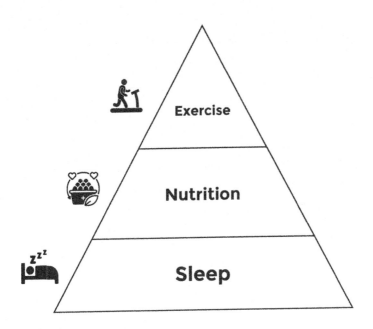

Therefore, the three foundational areas to maximize our energy are sleep, nutrition, and exercise. Each of these energy areas holistically and directly affect our energy edge - how much presence and power we bring to our days. When we intentionally and consciously improve and focus on each of these core health areas, we can generate the most energy. By following the techniques and strategies laid out in this book, you'll begin to *develop the awareness* that when you sleep better, you eat better and move and live more.

The Sleep Pyramid ™

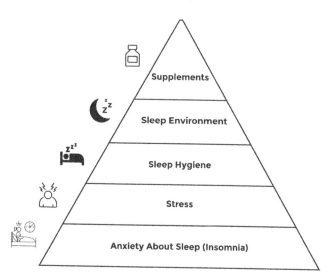

The sleep pyramid™ is a simple visual guide to what key areas should be focused on and in what order to improve one's quality of sleep.

Each of these sleep elements can have either a positive or negative effect on our sleep, and depending on what your unique sleep challenge is, it will indicate which area you should focus on first.

Many people make the mistake of focusing only on the 'seen' tangible areas to fix poor sleep such as taking sleep supplements, adjusting one's sleep environment, and practicing good sleep habits. What they fail to realize is the problem lies in the 'unseen.' **The real root cause of the challenge to fall and stay asleep is stress!** Not understanding this can become very frustrating and confusing and seem like the harder they try to sleep the worse they do. For example, they attempt the sleep shotgun supplement approach, which is trying many different types of sleep supplements such as valerian, CBD, kava kava, melatonin, 5-HTP, etc. Then after trying several different sleep supplements, they usually resort to adjusting their sleep environment, setting up blackout shades in their bedroom, wearing an eye mask and earplugs, and purchasing a new mattress. Then they may try cleaning up their sleep habits such as avoiding blue light from devices, eating and exercising earlier in the day, and maybe even listening to relaxing music, sleep hypnosis recordings, or practicing a bedtime meditation.

To be clear, everything I just said can and usually does support sleep quality, but not for someone with insomnia. The foundation for really increasing sleep quality is learning to master stress and practicing stress mastery techniques throughout the day. Let's explore some of these techniques now.

A great night's sleep happens as soon as you wake up!
Your decisions throughout the day will determine
the quality of your sleep at night.

Stress - The Great Sleep Disruptor

Stress is an inescapable part of our everyday lives. Stress can improve our sleep, health, energy, relationships, careers, and lives or destroy them. From the moment we wake up to the moment our head hits the pillow each night, we experience constant stress. We can't escape stress (even though we try), so we must learn how to master it. Mastery happens when we learn something and consistently implement it in our lives.

But what is stress? Stress can be defined as our bodies' and minds' responses to any demand, real or imagined, positive or negative. It's important to understand that not all stress is bad. Complimentary stress or *eustress* is the kind of stress that can have positive effects, such as exercising or studying for a test. Mostly, we feel stress whenever there is a challenge or a change in our life.

Stress, when understood and mastered, can be hugely beneficial. It can help us get things done, increase our creativity, and even enhance our performance.

For this book's purpose, we will be exploring complementary chronic mental stress, which makes up about 60-75% of our daily stress. This type of stress has very little benefit and comes from mainly how we think and the meaning we apply to our thinking. It's that feeling of your life being out of control and the perception that there are problems in your environment that you have no control over. It's the never-ending onslaught of emails, phone calls, text messages, bills, 'have-tos,' and 'to-dos.'

In today's fast-paced world, we all feel pressured to perform, handle more, and always be *on*. As a result, many of us have forgotten how to turn *off*, which is why we have trouble either getting or staying asleep each night.

We are overworked, overweight, overwhelmed, and consistently under-slept, all of which compound the adverse effects of stress in our daily lives. When we feel stress (whether it's real or perceived), our bodies' fight-or-flight (think survival) response is activated, triggering an increased heart rate, heightened muscle preparedness, sweating, and alertness.

All of these responses help protect us in dangerous or challenging situations but contribute to disease when left in the 'on' position for too long, which is what happens when we don't know how to release it from our mind-body system.

Unmastered chronic stress can have devastating consequences for our health. It's linked to just about every disease: obesity, type 2 diabetes, high blood pressure, cardiovascular disease, strokes, and Alzheimer's, to name a few.

According to the National Institute of Mental Health, it has been estimated that **75% to 90% of all doctor's office visits are for stress-related ailments and complaints.** We live in the middle of a stress epidemic, which contributes to the *lack of sleep* epidemic.

The World Health Organization stated that stress is the epidemic of the 21st century, and it's costing us big time. According to Gallup Research, only 30% of us are engaged and performing to our full potential, and almost half of us struggle to balance work and life.

When we don't learn how to release stress, our performance and ability to contribute our best to our families, organizations, and communities suffers. Unmastered stress is the number one performance killer and a thief of energy and joy. Unfortunately, we were never taught how to manage stress, let alone master it. We learned how to manage stress by those who didn't know how to manage their own.

We learned ineffective, counterproductive ways of managing stress, which can be summed up in three ways:

1. Lashing out in anger or frustration, which creates a loss of relationships.
2. Zoning out with T.V., movies, social media, or work, which can create a loss of time.
3. Numbing out with food, alcohol, and other drugs, which creates a loss of health.

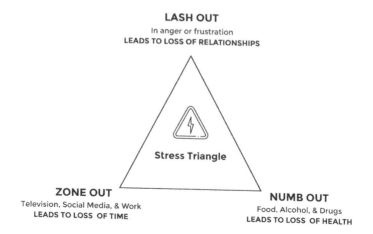

LASH OUT
In anger or frustration
LEADS TO LOSS OF RELATIONSHIPS

Stress Triangle

ZONE OUT
Television, Social Media, & Work
LEADS TO LOSS OF TIME

NUMB OUT
Food, Alcohol, & Drugs
LEADS TO LOSS OF HEALTH

The stress triangle is how most of us have learned to deal with stress, and it's creating so much of the unnecessary suffering in our lives.

Hopefully, at this point, you are wondering how do I become a master of my stress?

The first step to stress mastery is what I call creating 'stress awareness.' It's identifying your unique stress blueprint or how you deal with stress.

Simply put, a stress blueprint is a pre-set program of how we handle stress which includes a combination of thoughts, feelings, beliefs, and actions about real or perceived stress. It's our default-learned stress pattern.

How do you currently manage your stress? Do you lash out in anger and frustration? Zone out with work, T.V., shopping, surfing the web, or video games? Or numb out with eating too much food, drinking too much wine, or smoking? What's your stress pattern of choice?

The next step is learning to check-in, rather than check-out. This requires us to take a good look in the mirror and be honest with ourselves, even if we don't like what we see at the moment. This step can be uncomfortable because we have to be honest and identify the unhealthy ways we currently deal with stress.

The third step is implementing new strategies and tools to change our current stress blueprint. To do this, we must make stress mastery practices a non-negotiable part of our everyday lives. This takes a commitment but will allow us to retrain the parasympathetic relaxation response or, as I like to say, learn to switch off again.

Choosing to let go of self-chosen stressors, practicing mindfulness and meditation, cultivating authentic connection and community, and getting support from a coach or therapist allows us to live in higher efficiency. We can then tap into higher levels of natural energy to perform at an even higher capacity. It also allows us to get the much-needed sleep we need to do it all again the following day. We can't escape stress, which is why it's essential to learn how to self regulate and release it. To regulate stress, you have to find the strategies best suited to your needs and personality. This process takes time and requires openness and commitment.

One of the frameworks I use to help my clients rewire their stress blueprints is called the Release Method. The first step in the Release Method is to recognize that you are feeling stressed and Identify the root cause. What is the thought or belief that creates tension, tightness, and constriction in your body? Is the threat real or imagined?

The second step is to feel the stress. This is the part most of us want to skip because we're addicted to being comfortable; however, without feeling the pressure, it's much harder to release it. So, identify where you are holding the tension in your body. Usually, we feel stress in our neck, shoulders, stomach, face, or lower back.

The third step is to choose to *release it* by choosing to rest, recharge, or reset. Let's explore now how to rest, recharge, and reset.

Rest

Resting involves permitting ourselves to slow down and simply taking a few deep breaths. Unfortunately, because this is so easy to do, it's also easy not to do. Resting could also involve taking a short 20-minute recharge nap, taking a brisk walk, listening to a great song, or doing something that allows our body and mind just to slow down a bit.

Slowing down is the key to resting because when we experience stress, things seem to speed up, our minds race, our hearts race, and we kind of feel like we are in a race, but we are only in the race if we choose to be. Slowing down allows the energy to settle. Try this the next time you feel like you're rushing through your day or week: just slow down and take five deep breaths! When it feels like life is one emergency after another, consciously choose to slow down.

It helps to realize that doing nothing is doing something. The first time I understood this simple concept, it changed my life. I had adopted the hustle and achieve mentality when I opened my first business in college. I was going to school full time, then working with clients immediately after, and studying every second in between. I began to feel like a robot. I was exhausted and not prioritizing sleep or self-care, and it took its toll on me mentally and physically. I thought I didn't have the time to slow down, and I didn't have time to do *nothing* (which is another way of saying meditate, pray, or create intentional silent time). I developed the belief that I didn't deserve to rest until everything was done until the inbox of things to handle, accomplish, and do was empty. But I quickly discovered that this isn't a sustainable or joyful way to live. I found that I didn't need anything to experience the feelings of joy, peace, acceptance, and fulfillment that I was seeking through my constant doing. We are not human *doings*; we are human *beings*. It's so important to remember this and so easy to forget.

Slowing down helps us gain a much-needed perspective to make better decisions and choose things that are more in alignment with our values. Slowing down takes practice, and you may have massive resistance around it, especially if you are a Type A go-getter, hustling, high achiever. Slowing down is especially challenging when you are addicted to your stress hormones adrenaline, noradrenaline, and cortisol. Yes, that happens. You can become (and many of us are) addicted to the *high* you feel from your stress hormone supply.

Another critical insight to connect with is genuinely understanding why we may feel we are always rushing around. Maybe you identify being busy with being needed or important. Perhaps you feel like you haven't reached your goal or potential and don't deserve to rest until you do. Or maybe you feel that you haven't accomplished enough and that you don't deserve to rest until you achieve more. These are some common patterns I see when I work with high achievers with sleep challenges. I always remind them that the reason we do anything or want to achieve any goal is about how we think it's going to make us feel once we accomplish it. Life is all about feeling and meaning, and when we learn how to feel more and how to apply meaning in ways that are productive vs destructive, we have an advantage in the game of life and can leave the day behind us to sleep more soundly each night.

Recharge

Recharging involves implementing a consistent daily practice such as meditation that helps increase stress awareness and clears stress out of our body and mind. **Recharging is something we should not only do when we feel stressed, but every day to better prepare for stress**. You don't train for a marathon a week before the race. You train months in advance. So even when life seems calm and relaxed, stress awareness and mastery training are vital, because life always has a way of throwing us curve balls to help us grow.

Meditation retrains the body's parasympathetic nervous system to be able to turn on and off when appropriate. We must teach our bodies how to relax again, and meditation is a fantastic method to do just that. Meditation also just so happens to make us smarter, more creative, present, loving, and kind. You can think of meditation as going to the gym in your mind. The more you train, the stronger and better you get at it. When you practice meditation and mindfulness, you become more aware of your thoughts and have more control over which thoughts you pay attention to and which to let go of. You have the experience of separating yourself from your thoughts. Meditation is one of the simplest, yet most profound, life-changing gifts you could give yourself each day.

Meditation isn't just for monks. It's for anyone who wants to sleep better, perform better, be more creative, experience more happiness and joy, and feel more deeply. There are hundreds of great books on the scientifically proven benefits of mindfulness and meditation. Yes, it takes time (just 10 minutes a day of consistent meditation has shown incredible benefits). You may have to invest in learning how to do it, but let me ask a simple question: Are you willing to recharge and reset for just 1% of the day to make the other 99% better?

I hope you answered, *yes*.

Several great apps teach simple and effective meditation and mindfulness techniques. One of my personal favorites and one I often recommend is called *Head Space*. Another app I love and use every morning is called *Waking Up*. There are also excellent courses like Transcendental Meditation and Vipassana Meditation training that you can attend to learn highly effective techniques that have been used for thousands of years.

Reset

Resetting involves prioritizing time to play, ideally doing something active and fun with people you love. I don't know about you, but sometimes I take myself way too seriously. This constricts the fun and joy out of life. As children, we used to play, laugh, and imagine pretty much all day long, but as we become adults, life can seem much more serious. Play, laughter, and the use of our imagination become less frequent. Yes, there's a time and place to get serious, but more often than not, we way overdo it on the serious to fun spectrum, especially as we age and take on more responsibilities.

Laughter is medicine for the soul and is an incredible way of releasing stress and tension. Laughter triggers the release of endorphins, the body's natural feel-good chemicals. Endorphins promote an overall sense of well-being. Laughter has been found to strengthen our immune system, boost mood, diminish pain, and protect us from the damaging effects of stress. Laughter may even help us live longer.

Norwegian researchers reported findings from a 15-year study on the link between sense of humor and death among 53,556 women and men in their country. Using a validated questionnaire and examining death from specific conditions (heart disease, infection, cancer, and chronic obstructive pulmonary disease), they found that for women, high humor scores were associated with a 48% less risk of death from all causes, a 73% lower risk of death from heart disease, and an 83% lower risk of death from infection.

Nothing works faster or more dependably to bring our mind and body back into balance than a good laugh. By seeking out more opportunities for humor and laughter, we can improve our emotional health, strengthen our relationships, find a greater sense of happiness, and relieve physical tension and stress from our bodies, which leads to better sleep. What's also fantastic about laughter is that it's fun, free, and easy to use.

Setting an intention to laugh more and seeking opportunities to infuse some humor into our days is an incredible way of resetting.

Resetting also includes seeking and creating positive, authentic connections and community. In longevity studies, connection and community have proven to be the most influential factor for human health and longevity. If we feel lonely and isolated, our mental health suffers. And those with mental health challenges are more likely to suffer from insomnia or other sleep disorders. Plus, life is simply better when we have people we care about to share it with.

Resetting could also take the form of a weekend getaway once per month or at least once per quarter. It could be a stimulus reset, such as doing a weekend digital detox (no phone, computer, or T.V.), or taking that much-needed vacation.

Unfortunately, knowing better doesn't always lead to doing better. Knowledge isn't power, inspired action is. Taking inspired action is what creates change. Deciding to master our stress allows us to thrive versus simply survive, and it's worth the effort. Ultimately, becoming a master of stress takes commitment, time, and focus, yet it yields improved sleep, energy, joy, creativity, meaning, and purpose. Choosing to become the master of our stress is a lifelong practice. We will all experience loss, pain, and stressful events in our lives, so preparing now for these stressful events is one of the greatest gifts you can give yourself and your loved ones.

Stress and Sleep - A Vicious Cycle

It is no surprise that stress affects our sleep quantity and quality. When we are stressed or worried about something, it can seem almost impossible to quiet our minds long enough to drift off. I hear this all the time working with clients, "Devin, I just can't seem to turn my mind off at night. How do I turn my mind off?" With a mind that won't turn off, before we know it, it's 4:00 am and we still haven't fallen asleep; and, if we finally do drift off, we tend to toss and turn all night and have dreams about all the things we are worried about. This restless, unrefreshing sleep causes us to barely function the next day and to become even more stressed over not being as productive or creative as we'd hope to be. Research has shown us that stress and sleep are bidirectionally linked, meaning that the more stress you experience, the lower quality of sleep you get, and the lower the quality of sleep you get, the more stress you experience. This not-so-fun *sleep and stress* feedback loop can become what I call the "sleep paradox," which means that the more you try to sleep, the more elusive sleep becomes.

How do you turn off your mind at night to get to sleep and get out of this stress and sleep paradox?

It starts with creating space (I call this creating a "bed buffer") to allow your body and mind to unwind from the day's events. Just like you would prepare a baby or toddler for bed by bathing them, singing to them, rocking them in a rocking chair, and reading them a bedtime story, we must have a routine that we do each night to help us leave the day's wins and losses behind us. We will go into greater detail on how to do this in Part 3: Supporting Sleep.

Sleep and Mindfulness

Unfortunately, our mind doesn't work like a light switch. (Wouldn't it be nice if it did?) It doesn't just turn off. It never turns off even when we are asleep, which is one reason why it's essential to have a mindfulness practice. Practicing mindfulness trains us to become aware of our thoughts and the space in between them. The truth is, most of our lives we spend lost in thought. That is, we think, without knowing that we are thinking. This puts us at the mercy of whatever thoughts arise, and because of evolutionary survival programming the thinking is often in some form of, "is this safe?" Our mind is always looking for what's not right. Our mind becomes the theater of our worries, doubts, and fears, which creates anxiety and regret. Mindfulness is a way to break the spell and wake up to the beauty of the present moment. This doesn't come naturally, which is why we must practice it. I've found mindfulness to be one of the most effective and powerful techniques in helping clients naturally solve insomnia. I've worked with people who have "tried everything" and suffered from insomnia for decades, but now can fall and stay asleep all night from implementing particular mindfulness and coaching techniques. They say it's a miracle; I say it's mindfulness.

A new study published in 2015 in JAMA Internal Medicine included 49 middle-aged and older adults who had trouble sleeping. Half completed a mindfulness awareness program that taught them meditation and other exercises designed to help them focus on "moment-by-moment experiences, thoughts, and emotions." The other half completed a sleep education class that taught them ways to improve their sleep habits. Both groups met six times, once a week for two hours. Compared with the people in the sleep education group, those in the mindfulness group had less insomnia, fatigue, and depression at the end of the six sessions.

Another study published in Frontiers of Psychology in 2018 was conducted to investigate the effects of mindfulness training on insomnia and sleep quality in individuals with fibromyalgia (a chronic pain condition characterized by localized pain spots and prolonged generalized body pain). The experimental group was taught a specific mindfulness meditation technique over seven weeks. The results showed that compared to the control condition (the group who did not participate in the mindfulness program), the mindfulness intervention effectively reduced insomnia and improved sleep quality.

Why does mindfulness practice work so well for supporting sleep? It helps us improve our ability to see things as they are and gain much-needed perspective during challenging times. One of the most effective and straightforward mindfulness meditation tools is focusing on our breath. Intentionally breathing can shift both the mind and body in remarkable ways, because our breath is the anchor between the body and the mind. Using your breath to relax and release, rather than resist and persist, is a handy tool for finding balance in the brain and body.

Sleep Experiment

Take action: create a bed buffer.

Create a clear transition from your day to your night with a simple bed-time wind-down routine.

Try bed breathing:

Inhale through your nose slowly down into your diaphragm (stomach area) for a count of 4. Hold for a count of 7. Exhale from your mouth for a count of 8. Repeat this breathing cadence at least 12 times, which is the minimum amount of breaths that have been shown to activate the parasympathetic rest and digest response, or until you are relaxed or asleep.

Try taking energy breaks:

Experiment with taking 5-10 minute 'energy breaks' every 45-60 minutes throughout the day. Schedule these energy breaks in your calendar and stick to them. An energy break could involve walking up and down the stairs or around the building a few times. It could be as simple as bouncing up and down for a few minutes while taking several deep breaths. The best energy breaks include movement, drinking water, listening to upbeat music, and being outdoors to get fresh air and sun. Depending on your situation, do what is available to you. It will make all the difference at the end of the day when you try to shift out of work mode and into sleep mode!

How Sleep Affects Our Emotions

Think about the last time you had an emotional outburst. Maybe at work? On the road? With your spouse? With your kids? Chances are this happened because you were tired. When we are deprived of sleep, we're more likely to overreact to situations that usually wouldn't rattle us so much. If you have ever seen a 2-year-old who has skipped a nap, you can see a version of how we all react to sleep deprivation in terms of our emotions. Unfortunately, this is compounded by the fact that we don't usually notice this amplification of our emotional reactions. It's kind of like being buzzed on alcohol and thinking that you're okay to drive, when everyone around you can see you're not. The only person who can't see it is you.

Sleep plays such a critical role in our relationships. Getting the sleep we need acts as an emotional first aid. When we get the sleep we need, our brains are better able to process emotions and emotional events. We make better decisions and tend to be more patient. We have a greater ability to listen and concentrate when we're well-rested (all components of a healthy relationship).

An interesting example of this was found in a study on sleep and couples. The basics of the study were that one of the partners would get the normal amount of rest and the other partner would be deprived of two hours of sleep. Then after spending the day together, the couples were interviewed and asked to rate their partners on how they performed that day. They were asked about communication, connection, emotions, and mood. Interestingly, both partners rated the other as performing below their average. It didn't matter which partner was sleep deprived. It decreased the enjoyment of both partners equally. They both reported that their partner was less present, less connected, less communicative, and less fun as they usually were.

Other sleep and couples' studies have shown that men were more likely to fight with their wives after a night of disturbed sleep. I've personally experienced this in my relationship. On an occasional night when I don't sleep well, the little things that don't matter seem much more irritating. Another study conducted by Amie Gordon from the University of California found that couples who reported poor sleep during a two-week period reported more daily marital conflict than those who got better sleep. I think we've all experienced this at some level and it's not earth-shattering news that a lack of sleep hurts relationships, but sometimes we may overlook this common-sense relational circumstance. Getting enough sleep allows us to express our emotions better, communicate more effectively, and give those we love our full presence, strengthening the relationship. Simply put, when we sleep well, we do well in our relationships.

Sleep Experiment

Take action:

Don't have emotionally charged conversations before bed and especially not while in bed. Save the serious discussions with your significant other for a day when you are more rested. And on the days that you don't get great sleep, communicate this to your partner, spouse, and coworkers that work closely with you. Let the people around you know what's happening. Despite how this may seem, being open and vulnerable by communicating what's going on with you brings you closer to those around you and helps them understand if your behavior is slightly off. This could seriously make all the difference in the quality of your relationships.

The Sleep and Purpose Connection

Do you feel you are living your purpose? Are you connected to why you are here? Do you feel like you are living an authentically expressed life? Are you living the life that you desire or living a life based on what others desire for you?

These are not easy questions to answer, but when we take the time to be honest with ourselves, these questions can be life-changing. Now, you may be wondering what answering these questions has to do with sleep. Well, how we think and feel is usually expressed in what we do and do not do, which dictates our results. For instance, if you feel like you are not living your purpose, have no idea why you are here, or feel you're living someone else's version of your life and have trouble sleeping, do you think that has something to do do with it? Leland Val Van De Wall says, *"The degree to which a person can grow is directly proportional to the amount of truth he can accept about himself without running away."*

We often treat the top-of-mind symptoms (such as sleep challenges) with top-of-mind solutions or what I call band-aids (sleeping pills, supplements, alcohol, marijuana, etc.). Getting to the root of our psychological suffering can be the one thing that truly frees us from all physical manifestations of dis-ease, including sleep challenges. **Finding deeper meaning and purpose in our lives and embracing the discomfort that comes along with choosing to live an authentic fully expressed life, a life lived on our own terms, I believe is a key foundational element to improving sleep quality, energy, and overall well-being** and this isn't just my opinion. A 2017 study conducted by Northwestern University on the relationship between having a sense of purpose in life and its impact on sleep quality found that those who felt their lives had meaning were 63% less likely to have sleep apnea and 52% less likely to have restless leg syndrome, as well as reported having high-quality sleep. *Helping people cultivate a purpose in life could be an effective drug-free strategy to improve* *sleep quality, particularly for a population facing more insomnia,* said senior author Jason Ong, an Associate Professor of Neurology at Northwestern University Feinberg School of Medicine in Illinois.

So then the question becomes, *how does one cultivate a greater sense of purpose and live a more authentic, fully expressed life?* It starts with asking yourself better questions, then creating space to answer them honestly. Getting support from a therapist, counselor, or expert coach can help accelerate this process. Also, giving back creates a greater sense of purpose and meaning in life. Donating your time, talent, or energy to a cause you believe in or to others in need helps create meaning in your life. Mindfulness practices that increase awareness (such as meditation) are also fantastic tools for cultivating more meaning and purpose. I envision a future where instead of doctors prescribing sleep pills as the first line of therapy, they prescribe activities such as cognitive behavior therapy and mindfulness to help people sleep.

PART 3

Supporting Sleep

The Food and Sleep Connection

People are fed by the food industry, which pays no attention to health and treated by the health industry, which pays no attention to food. - Wendell Berry

We are what we eat. How we look, feel, and perform all significantly depends on *what* we eat and *how* we choose to eat it. But just as important (or possibly even more important) is what we *avoid* putting into our bodies.

It's effortless to eat poorly in today's *convenience-is-king* world. We are surrounded by fast and convenient foods that are engineered to taste incredible (they are designed to be addicting), and though these foods may taste good, they are terrible for our sleep, energy, and health. **Knowing what to avoid eating is just as important as knowing what to eat, so let's explore what to eat less of.**

Today, most people are starving for nutrients because about 70% of our diet consists of processed, artificial, 'fake' foods. Processed foods are made with low-quality ingredients and are loaded with sugar, preservatives, and other chemicals to make them convenient and taste great at the expense of our health. Once, while dining at a healthy restaurant, I saw a sign on the wall that read, "you are what you eat. So don't be fast, cheap, easy or fake." Reading it made me laugh out loud at first, then I realized the powerful truth in it.

The truth is that most big food corporations don't care about our health. Instead, their main goal is to create products that are fast, cheap, easy and fake. They produce food that will have a long shelf life, that we'll continually buy, and that will make them a profit.

Processed foods negatively interfere with our sleep. Processed foods contain unnatural chemicals, usually lots of sugar, and create food cravings the next day. Eating processed foods loaded with sugar (which often happens late at night when we are tired or need a distraction) spikes our blood sugar and affects our ability to wind down and prepare our mind and body for sleep.

When we consume sugar, it releases 'feel-good' hormones which make it highly addictive. It's been found that sugar is eight times more addictive than cocaine. Yes, you read that correctly. I know from personal experience: Oreos were my drug of choice.

Sugar is the number one energy draining food on the planet, and it is estimated that the average American consumes up to 150 pounds of sugar per year. That's about a half a pound per person per day. Yes, you read that one correctly, too…a half a pound! Despite the research linking sugar to just about every disease (including cancer, diabetes, heart disease, and chronic inflammation), it's tough to avoid because it's hiding in everything, even 'healthy' foods.

Without getting too scientific, when you consume sugar, your body has to release a hormone called insulin from your pancreas to shuttle the sugar from your blood to your muscles. The more sugar you have in your blood, the more insulin needs to be secreted to remove the excessive amount out of your blood, which leads to what I refer to as the 'sugar rollercoaster.' When you go more than a couple of hours without sugar after regular consumption, you will notice a drastic fluctuation, not only in your energy levels but possibly even in your mood - feeling an increase in irritability and anxiety. This 'sugar rollercoaster' that most of us ride daily creates cravings for more sugar to boost our mood and energy levels, which it does for a short time. The 'sugar rollercoaster' is kind of like a rollercoaster that never ends…it's fun while we are on it, but eventually takes its toll on our sleep, energy, and health.

When we are sleep deprived, our bodies and brains crave high fat and high sugar foods to lower the stress hormone cortisol. This is why our appetite increases when we get poor sleep. Also, our metabolism begins to slow down because it's trying to conserve the resources that we have in our system. It's a survival mechanism.

As I mentioned before, a lack of sleep also affects our *hunger* and *full* hormones, ghrelin and leptin. Ghrelin, the hormone that tells us to eat, actually increases; and leptin, the hormone that tells our body that we had enough to eat, decreases. When we are sleep deprived, we have a bigger appetite and burn fewer calories, not a good combo if you're trying to maintain a healthy weight.

Just like coming off a drug, getting off the 'sugar rollercoaster' does have some short-term withdrawal symptoms. The following are typical symptoms of sugar withdrawal, which can last a few hours or even days.

- Feeling lightheaded
- Extreme sugar cravings

- Feelings of anxiety, depression, and stress
- Headaches
- Nausea
- Moodiness
- Fatigue
- Achiness

There are several things we can do to help reduce our cravings and prevent us from giving in. Whenever cravings do hit, you should first and foremost drink a glass (or more) of water. Frequently, we feel hungry when we're thirsty. Dehydration can be masked as a craving, causing us to start searching for something to quench our thirst.

Sugar: Sleep Destroying Food #1

Consuming sugar throughout the day has been shown to interfere with deep sleep, resulting in unrefreshing sleep and fatigue the next day. Often sugar cravings kick in when we are tired and fatigued. When we are tired, our willpower is at its lowest, and our bodies crave sugar the most, hence the late-night sugar cravings. To make things even worse, when you regularly consume sugar, the late-night sugar cravings become even stronger. Eating sugary snacks right before bed affects more than just your quality of sleep, it also contributes to weight gain.

We started to touch on the dangers of sugar already but now let's dive deeper into how sugar affects our sleep more specifically. To make sure you're not consuming hidden sugars in your food, begin reading all food labels and look out for sugar. Four grams of sugar is equal to one teaspoon. Try to visualize how much sugar that is when you see something with 10 grams or 30 grams of sugar per serving. Ask yourself, *is this food going to give me sustained energy or keep me on the sugar rollercoaster?*

A simple strategy to avoid sugar is to stick to the outside aisles of the grocery store. Just about everything in the middle of most stores is processed, which usually means it contains a significant amount of sugar and preservatives. If you are a recovering sugar addict like I once was, stop buying it and bringing it into the house. Just as an alcoholic shouldn't have alcohol in their home, a sugar addict shouldn't bring sugar into it. After you kick the sugar habit, you can slowly reintroduce sugar into your diet outside the house, such as when dining out and on special occasions like anniversaries and birthdays.

Dairy: Sleep Destroying Food #2

Wait, doesn't milk build strong bones? Despite what we've been led to believe that milk *does the body good*, the truth is we've been deceived. Even though dairy contains a substantial amount of calcium, the phosphorus and acidic nature of dairy impair calcium absorption and utilization in the body.

We've also been told to drink a glass of warm milk at night when we're having trouble sleeping since it contains the sleep hormone melatonin and a sleep amino acid tryptophan, which are known substances to help in sleep and relaxation. But a glass of milk before bed can create mucus and inflammation in our bodies, which can bring on snoring due to lactose intolerance that creates mucus and unclear airways.

Our bodies just weren't designed to digest milk regularly, especially pasteurized milk. What's really interesting is that the majority of humans naturally stop producing significant amounts of lactase (the enzyme needed to properly metabolize lactose - the sugar in milk) some time between the ages of two and five. It's normal for most mammals to stop producing the enzymes needed to digest and metabolize milk after being weaned.

It's much better for our sleep and health to get calcium, potassium, protein, and fats from other food sources, like whole plant foods (vegetables, fruits, beans, whole grains, nuts, and seeds).

Try This Sleep Experiment:

Experiment with eliminating dairy for two weeks and see how it affects your sleep and energy. That means eliminate milk, cheese, yogurt, and ice cream for two weeks to feel the difference. You should notice improvements in your sleep, improved mental clarity, digestion, energy, and you most likely will even lose weight. After two weeks, try slowly incorporating some dairy back into your diet and see how you feel. If you feel gassy, bloated, mucousy, and sluggish, you should avoid dairy. Many companies now make great tasting natural plant-based dairy alternatives made from nuts. Give them a try.

What about coffee and caffeine?

Caffeine is the most abused legal drug, which dramatically disturbs our sleep. Even drinking caffeine in the morning or early afternoon could be affecting your sleep, because caffeine has a half-life of six to eight hours (depending on how you metabolize it), meaning it's in your system for 12-16 hours.

Consuming caffeine is kind of like borrowing from Peter to pay Paul. It provides a perceived temporary surge of energy and focus, but where did that energy come from? Without getting too technical, caffeine essentially blocks receptor sites in the brain that tell us when we need to rest. This then causes the activation of the hormone adrenaline to be released, putting us in the fight-or-flight response, which puts more stress on our adrenal glands (which produce hormones that are vital to life).

Caffeine simply masks what's happening inside our bodies and isn't a sustainable energy source. Caffeine can also create physical dependency. It's addictive, and the withdrawal symptoms from caffeine begin within one or two days after you stop consuming it. Like most drugs, caffeine increases dopamine production (the feel-good hormone), thus helping to maintain the dependency, which is consumed daily by 90% of all adults in the U.S.

By relying on caffeine, you are essentially borrowing tomorrow's energy today, which is simply not sustainable. However, I do have some good news for all the coffee lovers reading this: A cup of coffee in the morning isn't going to blow out your adrenals and massively affect your sleep at night. But if you are drinking multiple cups and rely on coffee to get you through the day to be productive and alert, chances are that you have an unhealthy dependency, which is affecting your sleep quality.

Maybe you can, or you know someone who can, drink a coffee and then go to sleep. Depending on your genetics, caffeine does affect people differently. That said, most people consume caffeine to increase alertness, which is the opposite of what we need before bed. Throughout the day, we have a neurochemical called adenosine that builds 'sleep pressure' or the body's hunger for sleep. Caffeine blocks the adenosine receptor sites in the brain. Sleep studies show that caffeine interferes with restorative deep sleep and REM sleep. As long as we eat a healthy diet, regularly exercise, and get enough quality sleep, we shouldn't need any synthetic or artificial energy to stay focused and productive. Imagine having sustained all-day energy with no dips or jitters. This is what's possible when you increase your sleep quality and reduce caffeine consumption.

Try This Sleep Experiment:

If you are currently only drinking one coffee per day and it's just because you love the taste rather than relying on it to function, then awesome.

Just try not to drink it past noon. If you are relying on coffee to get you through the day, try replacing your afternoon cup with dandelion coffee, which is a caffeine-free herbal tea made from the root of the dandelion plant that tastes similar to coffee. You can also try replacing coffee with herbal or green tea, which contains much less caffeine than coffee.

What About Alcohol?

Similarly, studies show that alcohol, even though it can make us feel sleepy, actually disturbs our sleep quality. Alcohol makes it harder to fall into the deeper stages of restorative sleep, which is what we are all striving for more of each night. If you measure your sleep, you'll see how, after even just one drink, your sleep quality is disturbed. Many people use alcohol to manage stress and take the 'edge off' after a long day. Unfortunately, this habit affects our natural energy edge, but there are way more productive and healthier ways of managing stress outside of consuming alcohol, which we touched on earlier.

Foods That Improve Sleep

Now that we know what *not* to eat and *not* drink to improve our sleep quality, what *should* we be eating instead?

What's good for our health is also good for our sleep. Foods that help support our sleep are no different than foods that support our general health. A diet rich in organic nuts, seeds, legumes, fruits, vegetables, wild seafood, grass-fed animal protein, and whole grains supports a healthy body.

Eating real food, real slow, is an excellent way to remember what and how you should be eating. An easy way to distinguish real food from fake food is remembering this little saying, *good food goes bad*. Food is not meant to last for months and years. Real food is minimally processed (if at all), fresh, and free of preservatives and chemical additives. This usually means eating local and organic food. Consume food that is free of all the dangerous conventional farming practices and is as close to where it was farmed as possible.

High-quality food that's wild and organic fuels a healthy body and mind, boosts the immune system, and is usually much lower in calories.

High-quality foods include:

- Organic whole grains (preferably gluten-free grains like amaranth, brown rice, buckwheat, oats, and quinoa)
- Organic fruits and vegetables
- Organic nuts, seeds, and beans
- Superfoods like spirulina and chlorella
- Responsibly farmed (wild, grass-fed, organic) animal products

There is no one size fits all approach to a healthy diet. A term that Joshua Rosenthal, the founder of the Institute for Integrative Nutrition (the world's largest nutrition school), uses to describe this concept is *Bio-Individuality*. We each are unique, have different body and blood types, live in different locations, have different genetics, caloric needs, and life-styles, so how could one diet work for us all?

Interestingly, you may find that even eating particular healthy food doesn't seem to work with your unique body. Figuring out what foods work for your body can be a difficult process. However, the more in-tune and aware you become of how you feel based on the food you eat, the easier it is to determine what foods work best for you. By staying connected and aware of how your body responds to the foods you're consuming (both the healthy and unhealthy foods), you'll be able to discover what works best for you. **Learning to listen to your body is one of the most significant skills you can practice in supporting longevity and health.**

The most common food sensitivities are dairy products, gluten, soy, sugar/artificial sweeteners, eggs, corn, and peanuts. Be especially aware of how your body responds when eating these particular foods. Low energy levels, mental fog, and nasal congestion are all signs you may be sensitive to a food or could have a compromised digestive system, also known as leaky gut.

Choose to eat for sustained energy and pleasure. Often people have a misconception that to be vibrantly healthy, you need to only eat food that doesn't taste very good and that all food that tastes amazing drains your energy. Going to either extreme isn't healthy, and truthfully, you can make performance foods (foods that fuel our energy) taste just as good (if not better) than the food that drains your energy.

A great food philosophy that is simple and works is the 80/20 to 90/10 philosophy. This simply means that 80% of the food you choose to eat is from healthy performance foods and the other 20% is from non-performance foods. Below is just a snapshot of some of my favorite high-performance foods:

- Herbs and spices like turmeric, garlic, and ginger
- Wild fish and seafood (salmon, sea bass, cod, and steelhead)
- Organic whole eggs
- Grass-fed meats and organic chicken
- Organically grown grains like brown rice, buckwheat, and quinoa
- Beans like black beans, pinto beans, navy beans, chickpeas, and great northern beans
- Nuts like almonds, cashews, and walnuts
- Seeds like flax, chia, hemp, and sunflower
- Vegetables (spinach, kale, brussels sprouts, cauliflower, carrots, beets, peas, and squash)
- Fruits (raspberries, blueberries, strawberries, peaches, grapefruits, pomegranates, and blackberries)

Several foods have been shown to support quality sleep because of their unique properties; for example, tart cherry juice contains naturally occurring melatonin. Kiwi fruit is packed with the sleep-promoting nutrients serotonin and folate. Researchers at Taiwan's Taipei Medical University studied the effects of kiwi consumption on sleep. They found that eating kiwi daily was linked to substantial improvements to both sleep quality and sleep quantity. Salmon and fatty fish help regulate serotonin, pumpkin seeds relax the muscles, and hummus is high in tryptophan, which helps you feel sleepy. Additionally, almonds, walnuts, and turkey have also been shown to help induce sleep at night.

Green vegetables from both land and sea are the most potent health foods on the planet. Although they support our sleep, unfortunately, they are the least consumed. They are the most anti-inflammatory of all foods and often contain the most nutrients from any food group. They are also loaded with chlorophyll, which is the lifeblood of plants and provides blood purifying and energizing properties when consumed.

Chlorophyll helps support our red blood cells, which carry oxygen throughout the body. Oxygen is essential to energy. Green foods also contain high amounts of calcium, magnesium, and potassium, all of which are necessary minerals for high-quality sleep. Not surprisingly, most people are deficient in these essential minerals. Many studies have shown a correlation between consuming greens and the protection against major chronic diseases such as cancer, diabetes, and cardiovascular disease. This could be linked to the sleep-enhancing benefits of these power-packed foods.

Green foods include:

- Leafy greens: kale, spinach, bok choy, swiss chards, collard greens, mustard greens, lettuce, arugula, and mache
- Broccoli, peas, green beans, brussel sprouts, and asparagus

- Wheatgrass and barley grass
- Parsley, basil, and cilantro
- Sea vegetables: kelp, Irish moss, kombu, dulse, nori, and arame
- Algae: spirulina and chlorella

All the superfoods above are ultra-energy and performance-enhancing and can be found at a natural grocer.

Try This Sleep Experiment:

Eat a massive salad every day for lunch or dinner. One of the quickest and easiest ways to get more greens into your diet is by starting the day with a green superfood smoothie or supplementing with a whole food greens powder.[3] There is no better way to start the day than with a green smoothie or juice. Another excellent energy option is to replace your afternoon coffee with green juice.

Hydration and Sleep

And last, but far from least – drink water! Being adequately hydrated is essential for optimal brain and body performance. Our bodies are composed of approximately 60% - 75% water. If you are not drinking at least half of your body weight in ounces per day, it's time to start. The benefits of being adequately hydrated are immense. When you're properly hydrated, you'll experience more energy, a clearer mind, and generally just feel better.

Dehydration is a major cause of daytime fatigue and energy slumps. When we are not adequately hydrated, we can experience headaches, mood fluctuations, and loss of focus and memory. If we wait to feel

---

[3]   Visit www.sleepscienceacademy.com/sleepadvantage to learn more about the greens product
       I personally use and recommend.

thirsty, we are already dehydrated. Up to 75% of Americans are reportedly chronically dehydrated.

Dehydration can cause us to be tired during the day, and it can negatively affect our sleep as well. Going to bed even mildly dehydrated can cause leg cramps and cause your mouth and nasal passages to dry out, leading to snoring.

Try This Sleep Experiment:

Purchase a 34-ounce stainless steel or glass water bottle and begin each day drinking 16-34 ounces of fresh spring water before your morning coffee. Remember, a great night's sleep starts as soon as you wake up, and this simple hydrate routine will support your energy edge throughout the day. It's important to mention that drinking too much before bed can cause you to wake up and have to use the restroom.

Meal Timing

What you eat matters, but *when* you eat matters just as much when it comes to increasing the quality of your sleep. This is because eating food too close to bedtime doesn't allow your body to get into full repair mode (what it's designed to do during the night). When you consume food within 3-4 hours before sleep, those calories from the food must be digested. Most people don't know that digestion takes a lot of energy and time. Think about it: the digestive process is where you are turning *food* into *your body*! As I mentioned before, you are what you eat. What happens is that during the digestive process, your body sends blood and uses the energy that would have been otherwise used to repair damaged cells while sleeping to your stomach to digest your food.

Specifically, studies show that **eating too close to bedtime disrupts deep slow-wave sleep or delta sleep, which is the most restorative stage of**

sleep, which takes place during the first quarter of the night. Deep sleep is when our bodies repair and recover the most, and it's a critical sleep stage because it's when the cleaning up of damaged cells (cancer cells) occurs. It's during deep sleep when the body heals and recovers the most during the night.

Try This Sleep Experiment:

Here are a few best practices to follow when it comes to nutrition and increasing sleep quality:

- Eat light evening meals (eat a larger breakfast, medium-sized lunch, and light dinner)
- Eat your evening meals as early as possible (5-7 pm)
- Incorporate some healthy carbs at dinnertime (think sweet potatoes and green vegetables)
- Light movement after meals, such as a walk, to help digestion

Exercise to Improve Sleep

If there were a pill that had all the benefits of exercise, the whole world would be taking it. —Bob Butler

We are designed to move our bodies. Movement is medicine. I believe there is an important distinction between movement and exercise. Movement ideally happens throughout our day; for example, walking to the mailbox or to the office, taking the stairs, gardening, taking the kids in and out of the car, etc. Exercise is a set period of time devoted to intentional movement. Ideally, we have both movement and exercise scheduled daily.

The challenge is that in the world we live in today, it's commonplace to sit. We sit on our couches, sit in our cars, and sit at the office. Sitting isn't a natural body position, and it violates the law of physical renewal, which states that our bodies are in a constant state of growth and rebirth, and if we are not moving our bodies enough, we are violating this law. The more we violate this law, the faster we age and die. This is why we must move our bodies daily to continue to create strong muscles, bones, nerves, connective tissue, and cartilage. It's just not natural to sit in front of a computer for hours on end, yet many of us do just that and then wonder why we feel tired, have back pain, and have trouble sleeping.

We are designed to move, not sit!

There are so many benefits to incorporating a daily movement practice into our lives. Rarely, health professionals can all agree on something, but all health professionals agree that moving our bodies daily is essential to our health. Yet, so many of us still don't take the time to do it. Movement is one of those things that we all know we should do more of, but often don't do enough.

There is no one-size-fits-all approach to movement and exercise that works for everyone. To experience how good our bodies are designed to feel consistently over the course of our lives, we must have a personal movement plan or what I call a PMP. A PMP simply consists of how and when you move your body. It's personal because it considers your age, fitness goals, lifestyle, and personal health history and preferences. Your PMP will and should evolve as you progress through life.

To create a PMP, I recommend investing in a qualified health professional to design one for you. Having a proper plan in place and the proper instruction to execute that plan is really important, and unless you have a degree in exercise philosophy or kinesiology, leave this to the pros.

Does Exercise Help Us Sleep?

When you incorporate regular exercise into your health routine, you will notice a drastic increase in how you *feel and* how you *sleep* at night. When we expend more energy during the day, we spend more time in deep sleep at night. Deep sleep has countless benefits, including cell regeneration, physical restoration, an increase in immune function, heart health support, and stress and anxiety control. And, since stress is a primary cause of sleep issues and exercise is a potent antidote to stress and anxiety, it only stands to reason that exercise is a no-brainer to improve your sleep quality.

Plus, when we exercise regularly, it's almost as if our bodies force us to rest because we feel more tired, and our bodies naturally go into rest mode. When we are fatigued after exerting physical energy, we spend more time in deep restorative sleep, and for a longer period of time.

Sleep Experiment

Take action: There are so many amazing and fun ways to move our bodies. Here are just a few: pilates, yoga, swimming, weight training, walking, jogging, dancing, cycling, spinning, bodyweight training, sports, stretching, rebounding, interval training, functional training, cross-training, tai chi, and qi gong.

My number one rule for exercise is to keep it simple and consistent. I can't stress this point enough. I've found both personally and from working with clients over the past decade that when things are simple, it's much easier for us to stay consistent, which leads to faster and long-lasting results. Schedule daily movement and exercise into your day and treat it as the most important appointment of your day. I know from experience that if it doesn't live on the calendar, it usually doesn't happen. As I mentioned above, it really helps to have professional support in creating and executing a fitness routine, especially if you don't have a degree in exercise physiology.

Establishing A Sleep Ritual

Having a sleep ritual is one of the best ways to improve sleep quality each night. Our bodies and minds love routines and rituals.

If you follow the same routine every night, your body will recognize the trigger to begin the sleep process and automatically start shifting into a lower gear. A sleep ritual can include anything from taking a warm shower, doing some light stretching, 'brain dumping' into a notebook, meditation, reading, or practicing a simple breathing exercise.

But, let me emphasize that the best bedtime *sleep ritual* is the one that you will consistently do each night! It's all about taking consistent and intelligent action.

It's so important to continually experiment to find what works best for you right now. Routines and rituals should evolve as you evolve. Once you discover something that works for you, do it with consistency and make it a habit.

Here is a sample of what an ideal healthy bedtime ritual could look like:

9:00 pm - Turn off all electronics (phone, tablet, television)
9:15 pm - Write out the day's wins and appreciations, and do a brain dump
9:30 pm - Take a warm/cold shower
9:45 pm - Lightly stretch or foam roll while listening to relaxing music
10:00 pm - Sip herbal tea and read a good book
10:15 pm - Slide into bed and turn the lights out

Try This Sleep Experiment:

Set a 3-2-1 alarm. Just like you may use an alarm to wake up, set the alarm to begin your evening sleep ritual. This acts as a trigger to begin the bedtime wind-down process.

3...2...1 sleep. This was shared with me from one of my mentors, and I love it:

3 hours before bed - No more food; four hours would be even better!
2 hours before bed - No more work (email, social media, news, texts, etc.).
1 hour before bed - No screen time (T.V., phone, iPad, etc.). Start your sleep wind-down ritual.

Create Your Sleep Sanctuary

Make It Cool

The bedroom is the most important room in the entire house. It's where we spend a third of our life and where intimacy happens. And if our bedroom is the most important room in our home (and it is), that means that our bed is the most important piece of furniture we own.

In case you couldn't tell by now, I am a huge fan of optimizing things. I love making things better and feeling the effects of making inspired, intelligent adjustments to my environment. If there is one room in your home that you should optimize, which simply means *make it better*, it's the bedroom.

So, what does an optimized bedroom look and feel like? For starters, it's cold, clean, and clear of clutter. Why cold? We need a drop in our body temperature by two to three degrees Fahrenheit to initiate sleep. This is why, as you may have experienced, it's always easier to fall and stay asleep in a cool versus hot room. Furthermore, regulating your body temperature overnight is key for optimizing sleep quality. If you can keep your bedroom set between 65-68 degrees, that allows your body to cool to the optimal sleep temperature.

Sleep Experiment

Take action: Drop the temperature in your home before bed to between 65-68 degrees Fahrenheit and wear wool socks to bed. Making your feet warm during the night causes something called 'vasodilatation,' which is the dilation of the blood vessels. Vasodilatation of your hands and feet help to lower the core body temperature, inducing sleepiness. Wait... why wool? Wool is naturally anti-stick and if you wear cotton socks to bed, your feet may begin to smell. You can also try taking a warm or hot shower before bed to help get your body temperature down as well.

Keep It Clean and Clear of Clutter

You may not think it's important, but surprisingly, keeping your bedroom neat and tidy has been shown to minimize feelings of anxiety and can calm our mental energy. Similarly, crawling into a made bed with clean sheets will make all the difference. If you make your bed a trigger for sleep (meaning not for watching TV or eating), your mind will automatically be trained that bed equals sleep when you crawl in. Having clean bedsheets, pillowcases, and blankets are integral to a great night's sleep and an optimized bedroom. Would you wear sweaty, drool-stained, dirty clothes to work? Probably not, because you wouldn't feel great in them. The same goes for bedding. Change your sheets at least once per week. Speaking of sheets, I'll never forget my first experience sleeping with bamboo sheets. All my life I had slept with cotton sheets. I had read and heard how bamboo had a silky feel and kept the body cool and how it made for great bedsheets, but I didn't think much of it until I was given a pair as a wedding gift. Wow, talk about a bedtime game-changer! Once you go bamboo, you don't go back. They are ultra-soft and truly help to keep you cool throughout the entire night, and in my opinion, are worth the investment. Investing in high-quality, comfortable bedding, pillows, and mattress isn't only a luxury, it's a necessity if you desire to have a great night's rest.

Sleep Experiment

Take action: Upgrade your bedding, pillows, and mattress. [4]

Make it Dark

Biologically, our bodies are designed to synchronize with natural light, as this is what we have naturally done since the beginning of time. It wasn't until quite recently that we have been exposed to synthetic light sources from light bulbs, TV, iPads, and smartphones, which have greatly affected our circadian rhythm, thereby affecting our sleep quality.

Our bodies are still designed to respond to light cues, including bright light in the morning, natural light throughout the day, dark nights, and waxing and waning of the moon. Remember our circadian rhythm is our 24-hour physiological biological clock that is regulated by the sun, moon, and temperature.

Of course, in an ideal world we would continue to experience lighting as our bodies were evolutionarily designed, such as sleeping under the stars and consistently absorbing the sun and natural light throughout the day. We would wake and sleep around the same time every day, as dictated by the earth's natural rhythms.

---

[4]   For my personal recommended mattresses and bedding brands, visit
      www.SleepScienceAcademy.com/sleepadvantage

Instead, today we spend more time indoors, exposed to unnatural and blue lighting, drastically affecting our circadian rhythm, sleep quality, and overall health.

Darkness

A complete lack of light - actual cave-like darkness - is essential for optimal sleep. We need natural light and natural darkness to help our bodies synchronize our circadian rhythm; otherwise, we will put ourselves in a period of limbo between night and day. Of course, the earlier in the evening we can follow the cue to sleep, the better our sleep will be, and the greater we will benefit. Constant light (or darkness) doesn't allow for our bodies and minds to receive the signals we were evolutionarily designed to receive.

Try This Sleep Experiment:

Get black-out shades in your bedroom or wear a sleep mask to keep it dark. As the sun begins to set, begin turning down the lights in your home. If you really want to go the extra mile, replace your LED lights with good dimmable incandescent bulbs.

Blue Lighting

Blue lighting (light from televisions, computers, phones, etc.) has the greatest negative impact on our ability to experience quality sleep at night. Blue light during the day has a lesser effect than at night, of course. While it's a tall order, it is recommended that we experience no blue light for three hours before we plan to go to sleep. If that's not possible, install a blue-light-blocking application like F.lux or Iris or wear blue-light-blocking glasses. Ideally, at least an hour before you'd like to be asleep, keep away from blue light. This will make all the difference.

Seasonal Affective Disorder (SAD) is a form of depression that is triggered by a lack of natural light, which is most apparent during the wintertime. I actually suffered from SAD growing up in Philadelphia as a teenager. Each winter, I would get the 'winter blues.' This would happen because I would wake up before the sun to go to mandatory morning basketball workouts, spend the rest of the day in a classroom, and then go to basketball practice after school only to return home in the dark. This would go on for the entire basketball season, and each year I would begin to feel depressed a few weeks into the season. My concerned Mom eventually started to research 'Winter Depression,' and we learned about SAD. She bought me a 'natural sunlight lamp,' and each night after basketball practice, I would sit in front of the light listening to the Beach Boys soundtrack, and it helped me. The long winter months without sun eventually led me to attend a college in the 'sunshine state' Florida, and I haven't had SAD since.

Many of our sleep issues can be alleviated by just getting more natural light and complete darkness as we were evolutionarily meant to get. If you experience any of the below issues, the culprit could be a result of not getting enough sunlight:

- Not hungry in the morning
- Feeling hungry late at night
- Binging
- Cravings for carbs
- Sleep disturbances
- Moodiness
- Lack of motivation
- Issues with digestion

While there are many things one can do to improve our exposure to natural light, the most important thing is exposure to bright light early in the morning and getting more hours of complete darkness at night.

Try This Sleep Experiment:

As soon as you wake up, get 15 minutes of natural sunlight. If you wake up before the sun, experiment with using a lightbox during the same time frame in the morning and taking a walk at lunch. If you live in a place that has cold, dark, long winter nights, consider investing in a sun lamp to expose yourself to more light. The key is consistency.

Everything You Need to Know About Sleep Supplements

Before we get into the details about the best supplements that can help support your sleep, it's crucial to understand a few things about the supplement industry and sleep.

Supplements can be incredible when you use them in addition to a healthy lifestyle. What is a healthy lifestyle? It entails managing stress, finding purpose in your work, drinking clean water, eating organic high-quality food, exercising, and cultivating quality relationships.

Please don't make the mistake of thinking that taking a sleep supplement will make a difference if you are currently eating a poor diet, not healthily managing your stress, drinking excessive alcohol, and not practicing good sleep habits.

We have been conditioned by society to always look for the quick fix, the silver bullet. Wouldn't it be nice if only it was that easy? Unfortunately, very seldom do these quick-fix silver bullets (aka sleep supplements) address the root cause (what needs to be addressed) to have a sustainable outcome. Like the pharmaceutical industry, the supplement industry has taken advantage of this quick fix conditioning.

Have a headache? Take this…

Can't get it up? Take that…

Want to lose weight? Just take this fat burner…

Can't sleep? Pop this…

…and on and on.

Like me, maybe you've discovered through your own health journey, experimentation, and education that everything in life comes down to quality and knowing what, when, and how to take action.

There are literally thousands of sleep supplements on the market today, each promising to be the answer to your sleep problems. Here is the straight and honest truth: Some sleep supplements work, most of them don't. Unfortunately, there's also relatively limited research that investigates the direct benefits of sleep supplements because of a lack of funding. The sleep supplements that I'm going to be sharing with you are backed by research.

When you are considering taking a sleep supplement, you'll want to be clear that everything in the formula, every last ingredient, is sourced for purity, efficacy, and safety. That's step one.

This is because the supplement industry is virtually unregulated. What does 'essentially unregulated' mean? The Food and Drug Administration (FDA) mandates that dietary supplements sold to U.S. customers aren't mislabeled and don't contain banned substances, according to the Dietary Supplement Health and Education Act of 1994. That sounds great in theory, but here's the issue: The FDA doesn't evaluate the safety or label accuracy of supplement companies—they leave it to the manufacturers themselves to enforce. Of course, there is a gigantic economic bias for manufacturers to report their products as safe, even if they aren't correctly tested or safe.

This regulation strategy isn't working. According to a 2015 New York Attorney General investigation, four out of five herbal supplements don't have listed ingredients.

How can health-conscious supplement consumers avoid harmful toxins and ensure they're taking accurately-labeled supplements? Look for a supplement manufacturer based in the U.S. that performs third-party testing of their products.

Step two is finding a formula that is personalized to your unique sleep challenge. Your unique biochemistry, chronotype, health history, lifestyle, and sleep challenges are all factors to consider when deciding what sleep supplement is best for you. Personalization is always the best because we are all unique. What works for one person may not work for another. This is where it can get a bit tricky.

You'll also want to consider why you're taking a sleep supplement in the first place. If you have chronic insomnia (issues getting or staying asleep three days per week for longer than three months), ideally you need to first address the lifestyle issues that are actually causing the sleep problems. In this case, taking a supplement should really be your last consideration, not your first.

If you sleep fairly well and are looking to improve the quality of your sleep, supplements can play more of a role.

I believe in taking herbs and natural medicine. There is a place for sleep supplements, so let's talk about some of the most effective herbs, amino acids, vitamins, and minerals that help promote rest and relaxation.

Important Disclaimer: This is not medical advice, but it is information you can use as a conversation-starter with your health practitioner at your next appointment. Always consult your doctor or health practitioner before taking a supplement or making any changes to your existing medication and supplement routine.

Sleep Supporting Herbs

Cannabidiol (CBD): Supports falling asleep, staying asleep, and quality of sleep.

CBD, also known as hemp oil, is quickly becoming one of the most highly sought after and used sleep supplements in the world. Why? Because its benefits are finally being discovered and shared. It also just so happens to help alleviate three of the most common 21st-century health conditions:

1. Stress and Anxiety
2. Sleep Issues
3. Physical Pain

What is CBD?

Cannabidiol, or CBD, is a non-psychoactive chemical compound that's found in the cannabis plant. It is one of over 60+ different compounds present in cannabis. CBD is usually present in cannabis in high concentrations along with THC (the compound in cannabis that is psychoactive and makes you feel high).

How does it work?

In your body, you have what's called an endocannabinoid system (ECS), a complex cell-signaling system identified in the early 1990s by researchers exploring THC, a well-known cannabinoid. Cannabinoids are compounds found in cannabis. Interestingly, the ECS exists and is active in your body, even if you don't use cannabis.

Without getting overly scientific and complex, there are two types of cannabinoid receptors in the human body: CB1 and CB2. Both are naturally found throughout the body but are most common in the brain and immune system.

CB1 receptors are responsible for marijuana's psychoactive effects. These receptors affect sleep, memory, mood, appetite, and pain sensation. CB2 receptors have anti-inflammatory effects and are found in immune cells. CBD does have a high affinity and attraction for CB2 receptors, making it an excellent natural relaxant, anti-inflammatory, and immune system booster.

CBD supports sleep because it can help relax the body to prepare for restful sleep. As I mentioned, CBD also works as an analgesic—a pain reducer—in the body that supports those who have trouble sleeping from chronic pain.

According to studies, CBD can significantly support reducing insomnia symptoms and can increase overall sleep duration. In smaller doses, CBD can stimulate alertness and reduce daytime sleepiness, which is important for daytime performance and the strength and consistency of the sleep-wake cycle. This unique feature of consuming CBD can make dosing challenging. New research shows that it relieves anxiety without causing changes to healthy sleep-wake cycles.

Some common questions about CBD

Is CBD legal?

Unlike marijuana, CBD is legal in the USA. On February 7, 2014, President Obama signed the farm bill of 2013 into law, which defined industrial hemp as distinctly different from marijuana. It further states that as long as the cannabis Sativa plant has less than .3% THC, it qualifies as industrial hemp and is legal to be grown and sold in the United States.

Will CBD make me feel high?

CBD offers many of the same benefits of marijuana without the high because it contains only minimal, if any, amounts of THC tetrahydro-cannabinol (THC). It is entirely safe and nonaddictive when purchased from reliable quality sources.

Does CBD have any other benefits?

Studies have found that CBD can…

1. Relieve nausea and vomiting, making it a great digestive aid
2. Help control and reduce seizures
3. Help fight tumors and cancer cells, because it's a powerful antioxidant
4. Help relieve anxiety and depression
5. Calm and protect the nervous system
6. Promote relaxation and deeper sleep
7. Help reduce stress
8. Help relieve insomnia
9. Help reduce swelling and inflammation
10. Help relieve muscle and joint pain

What are the most popular uses of CBD?

Most people are using CBD as a natural alternative to help support anxiety, reduce physical pain, and promote relaxation to improve sleep. As mentioned before, it's also been proven to be a highly beneficial treatment for seizures and neurological conditions such as Multiple Sclerosis.

Which method of consumption is best?

CBD is extracted as an oil from cannabis or hemp plants and comes in various concentrations and forms. It can be consumed as an edible, in a capsule form, as a liquid tincture, vaporized, or sprayed into the mouth. It can also be used topically and absorbed into the bloodstream through the skin from an externally applied cream. Which product form you consume depends on why you are using CBD, how quickly you would like to experience the benefits, and your personal preferences.

- Vaporizing CBD is a fast way to get CBD into the body, usually within minutes.
- Consuming edibles, capsules, oil tinctures, or sprays usually takes 2-4 hours.
- Topically it takes 1-6 hours.

The best method of consumption depends on personal preference. The quality of the product and the number of milligrams are also factors to consider.

Does CBD have side effects?

CBD rarely has side effects when using the commonly recommended doses of anywhere between 2.5 mg to 1500 mg.

- However, studies have found possible side effects may include:
- Drowsiness
- Diarrhea
- Increases or decreases in appetite

Minus diarrhea, these side effects could potentially be beneficial depending on the reason you're taking CBD in the first place. Often CBD users are using CBD to help them get better quality sleep. The majority of studies currently available were performed for the treatment of epilepsy and psychotic disorders. Here, the most commonly reported side effects were tiredness, diarrhea, and appetite as well as weight changes. Compared with other drugs used for the treatment of these medical conditions, CBD has a better side effect profile. However, more clinical trials with a greater number of participants and more extended CBD administration are needed.

Is CBD addictive?

CBD is non-addictive and safe when you're getting your CBD products from a reputable source. Unfortunately, because the benefits of consuming CBD are becoming more and more known, many companies are flooding the CBD market with poor quality and ineffective products. You want to look for reputable companies that offer organically grown, full-spectrum, CO_2 extracted CBD.

Will taking CBD fail my drug test?

This is a common question, and the simple answer is 'no.' This is because legal CBD products contain no traceable amounts of THC (the chemical in marijuana that causes people to get high). However, consumers using substantial doses of CBD-rich hemp oil products above 1000-2000 mg daily could potentially have a false positive during initial screening due to other non-THC metabolites that may cross-react with the test. This is extremely rare.

How much CBD should I take? How do you dose CBD correctly?

There is no one size fits all or easy answer to this question. It really depends on several factors. First, it depends on the quality of the CBD product that you are using. Second, it depends on the reason you are using CBD. Are you using it to relieve pain, help you get to sleep, or to manage anxiety? Third, it depends on how much you weigh. Weight as a factor influences your metabolism, circulation, and health. However, everybody is different, so it's best to experiment with different dosages until you achieve the desired effect.

Intake Guidelines:

Start small – start with the smallest dose possible. Everyone reacts differently to various supplements, so it's important to become familiar with how your body responds. A good starting dose is 15-20 mg. In my experience, therapeutic relaxation effects are felt after consuming high-quality CBD in the dose range of 40-50 mg.

Size Matters – larger individuals may prefer a higher dose of CBD than smaller people. With CBD, you can easily scale up just a few mg at a time to meet your needs.

Consistency is key – using CBD consistently stimulates a healthy, functioning endocannabinoid system. As cannabinoids enter the system, your body becomes more sensitive over time.

*Consult with a medical professional if you have a serious medical condition. Always consult with a qualified healthcare professional before consuming CBD.

When is the best time to take CBD?

Again, it really depends on why you are taking it in the first place. It also depends on the method of consumption. Generally speaking, most people take CBD an hour to a few hours before bed to help improve their sleep. Those who take it to manage pain should take it in the morning, and those who take it to alleviate stress and anxiety can take it anytime throughout the day.

Where do I get high-quality CBD products?

As more scientific studies are released on the benefits of CBD, more and more products continue to hit the consumer market. You can purchase a wide variety of CBD products online and in some health food stores across the country.

As with all supplements, it's important to consider the quality, extraction, storage, and manufacturing methods before purchasing a product. Many supplements on the market today are ineffective and a complete waste of money because they simply aren't of quality ingredients or have poor extraction methods, making them ineffective at best.

When evaluating a CBD product or company, look for these marks of quality:

- Organically sourced
- CO_2 extraction method
- Third-party tested for impurities
- The manufacturer is both GMP (Good Manufacturing Practice) and PETA approved
- Whole plant extracted CBD - extracted from the stalk, flowers, and leaves - not just the stalk (full-spectrum hemp oil)

High-quality CBD is a great alternative to dangerous sleep medications and can help people fall and stay asleep throughout the night.

Lemon Balm - Helps you relax to fall asleep faster.

Lemon Balm is an herb, part of the mint family. It has been used medicinally for centuries to address sleep challenges. It has been found to help reduce anxiety, especially when combined with valerian root.

It has also been shown to decrease feelings of stress and tension, as well as decrease fatigue due to stress, while increasing calmness, thus supporting falling asleep quicker.

It's also been found to help support those suffering from insomnia, especially women during menopause.

Several studies show that lemon balm, when combined with other calming herbs (such as valerian, hops, and chamomile), has a very relaxing effect.

Intake Guidelines:

Many sleep supplements combine lemon balm with other sleep-promoting herbs. Lemon balm is usually consumed in either a capsule or liquid tincture form. A 300-600 mg dose has been shown to produce calming effects.[5]

---

[5] Visit www.SleepScienceAcademy.com/sleepadvantage to learn more about the sleep supplement brands that I recommend.

Valerian Root - Supports falling asleep more quickly, increases the quality of sleep, and increases amounts of nightly sleep.

Valerian root is sometimes referred to as 'nature's Valium' and has been used since ancient times to promote tranquility and improve sleep. It's an herb grown throughout Asia and Europe and is now also grown in the US, China, and many other countries. Valerian is one of the best-studied herbs for sleep. At least a dozen or more scientific studies have found valerian - used on its own or in combination with other herbs such as hops - to improve sleep. Research shows that valerian can help people fall asleep more quickly, improve the quality of sleep, and increase amounts of nightly sleep.

Valerian can also help ease the symptoms of insomnia, which are:

- Difficulty falling asleep
- Trouble staying asleep
- Waking very early
- Waking feeling unrefreshed

How it works:

Valerian contains valerenic acid which has been shown to inhibit the breakdown of GABA. This chemical messenger helps regulate nerve impulses in your brain and nervous system, which results in feelings of calmness and peace, similar to how both Valium and Xanax work. Evidence suggests that low GABA levels related to stress are linked to anxiety and low-quality sleep. Taking valerian root may reduce the amount of time it takes to fall asleep and improve sleep quality and quantity.

Intake Guidelines:

Most studies of people with sleeping difficulties have found between 400–900 mg of valerian extract to be a safe and effective dosage for sleep support. In general, it's recommended that users begin with the smallest suggested dose of valerian and gradually increase it until it has an effect.

For the best results, take it 30 minutes to two hours before bedtime. It has been found that valerian is most effective after taking it consistently for at least two weeks. It can be consumed as a tea, a tincture, or in capsule form and is often found in herbal sleep formulations.

Note: Valerian has a very strong odor that many people (myself included) find unpleasant. If you are not a fan of the stinky smelling tea, then look for valerian in pill form or in a tincture to avoid this smell.

Hops Flower - Supports falling asleep.

Historically, hops were a traditional medicine used as one of the herbs for sleep because of their calming, sedating, and hypnotic (sleep-inducing) effects. Hops also have a long history of use in herbal medicine, dating back to at least the 9th century in Europe.

Studies show that hops can boost GABA production, a calming brain chemical that promotes sleep. Hops also have mild sedative properties, and therapeutic doses of this plant lower body temperature, which contributes to drowsiness.

Hops may also be more effective when used in combination with valerian, this is because certain herbs work synergistically together to enhance the positive effects of each other.

Intake Guidelines:

Hops on its own: 300-500 mg. Valerian in combination with hops: 187-250 mg valerian, 42-60 mg hops.

Sleep Supporting Amino Acids

GABA (Gamma-Aminobutyric Acid) - Helps you fall and stay asleep.

GABA is an amino acid produced naturally in the brain. GABA functions as a neurotransmitter, facilitating communication among brain cells. GABA's significant role in the body is to reduce the activity of neurons in the brain and central nervous system, which has a broad range of effects on the body and mind.

By inhibiting neural activity, GABA facilitates sleep, reduces mental and physical stress, lowers anxiety, and creates a calm mood.

Think of GABA as the brakes of the brain. GABA is the body's most important inhibitory neurotransmitter, which lowers the activity of neural cells in the brain and central nervous system, supporting the brain and body to shift into a lower gear.

The body's own GABA activity is essential for sleep because it enables the body and mind to relax and fall and stay asleep throughout the night.

Studies show that low GABA activity in the brain has been linked to insomnia. In a study conducted by Harvard Medical School, GABA levels in people with insomnia were almost 30 % lower than those without sleep disorder. And these low GABA levels also corresponded to more restless, wakeful sleep. Interestingly, big-pharma sleep medications, including those with zolpidem (Ambien and others) and eszopiclone (Lunesta and others), target the body's GABA system to increase sedation and sleep.

As a natural chemical that the body produces, GABA's primary role is to diminish the activity of neurons in the brain and central nervous system, which puts the body in a greater state of relaxation and alleviates stress and anxiety.

Supplemental GABA may benefit sleep by aiding in the relaxation response and providing relief from mental anxiety and stress. There still remains much debate among scientists about supplemental GABA's effectiveness and whether it is able to cross the blood-brain barrier via the bloodstream. Although more research is still needed, GABA in supplement form may have other ways of relaxing the body and relieving stress, possibly through the gut microbiome.

Intake Guidelines:

The following doses are based on amounts that have been investigated in scientific studies. In general, it is recommended that users begin with the lowest suggested dose and gradually increase as needed.

For sleep, stress, and anxiety: 100-200 mg and higher doses, based on scientific studies. Individual dosing and length of use will vary.

GABA Interactions

High blood pressure, antidepressant, and neurally-active medications are commonly used medications and supplements that have scientifical-ly-identified interactions with GABA. People who take these or any other medications and supplements should consult with a physician before beginning to use GABA as a supplement.

5-HTP (5-Hydroxytryptophan) - Increases quality of sleep.

5-Hydroxytryptophan, commonly known as 5-HTP, is a by-product of the amino acid L-tryptophan. Our bodies don't make L-tryptophan naturally, rather we absorb this essential amino acid from the foods we consume, including chicken, turkey, eggs, fish, and pumpkin and sesame seeds.

5-HTP helps the body to produce more serotonin. Serotonin is a neurotransmitter that plays a key role in regulating mood and sleep-wake cycles. Healthy levels of serotonin contribute to a positive mood and outlook and also promote restful sleep. One important way that serotonin affects sleep is through its relationship with the sleep hormone melatonin. Melatonin is made from serotonin in the presence of darkness. Melatonin production in the body is triggered by darkness and suppressed by exposure to both natural and artificial light. With its ability to increase serotonin, 5-HTP supports a neurochemical process that can enable high-quality sleep and keep the body's biological clock in sync.

Supplementing with 5-HTP may help both shorten the time it takes to fall asleep and increase sleep duration. 5-HTP has also been found to support a positive mood and ease symptoms of stress and anxiety, which often interfere with sleep.

Intake Guidelines:

The following doses are based on amounts that have been investigated in scientific studies. In general, it is recommended that users begin with the smallest suggested dose and gradually increase it until it has an effect.

A range of doses from 25 mg to 500 mg and higher have been studied in scientific research for sleep problems, anxiety, depression, and stress.

L-theanine - Supports falling asleep.

L-theanine is an amino acid that is found in tea leaves. It was identified in tea by Japanese scientists in 1949. While tea is the most common dietary source for L-theanine, this compound is also found in some types of mushrooms. L-theanine promotes relaxation and facilitates sleep by contributing to a number of changes in the brain.

L-theanine boosts levels of GABA and other calming neurotransmitters such as serotonin and dopamine in the brain. L-theanine has also been shown to improve the quality of sleep—not by acting as a sedative, but by lowering anxiety and promoting relaxation.

L-theanine has been found to enhance alpha brain waves. Alpha waves are also present during REM sleep. L-theanine appears to trigger the release of alpha-waves, which enhances relaxation, focus, and creativity. Unlike valerian and hops, which have sedative effects, L-theanine promotes relaxation and stress reduction without sedating.

Interesting fact: L-theanine combined with caffeine can enhance cognitive performance. Studies show that combinations of L-theanine and caffeine can improve attention span, enhance the ability to process visual information, and increase accuracy when switching from one task to another. In combination with caffeine: 12-100 mg L-theanine, 30-100 mg caffeine.

Intake Guidelines:

The following doses are based on amounts that have been investigated in scientific studies. In general, it is recommended that users begin with the smallest suggested dose, and gradually increase until it has an effect. For sleep, stress, and other uses: 100 mg to 400 mg.

Glycine - Supports falling and staying asleep, as well as increases sleep quality (deep and REM sleep stages).

Glycine (also known as 2-Aminoacetic Acid) is an amino acid and a neurotransmitter. The body produces glycine on its own, synthesized from other natural biochemicals. This amino acid is found in high-protein foods, including bone broth, meat, fish, eggs, dairy, and legumes.

How does glycine support sleep?

Glycine helps lower body temperature. Glycine works to increase blood flow to the body's extremities, which reduces core body temperature. A slight drop in body temperature is a key part of the body's physical progression into sleep. Some studies suggest that supplemental glycine may help you move more quickly into deep, slow-wave sleep, as well as spend more time in REM sleep.

Glycine also increases serotonin levels, a hormone and neurotransmitter that significantly affects sleep and mood. Serotonin has a complex relationship to sleep. Among other things, serotonin is required to make the sleep hormone melatonin. In people who have difficulty sleeping or sleep disorders such as insomnia and sleep apnea, increasing serotonin levels can help restore healthy sleep patterns and encourage deeper, more restful, and refreshing sleep. Research shows oral glycine elevates serotonin, reduces symptoms of insomnia, and improves sleep quality. Other studies suggest it may help you bounce back to healthy sleep cycles after a period of disrupted sleep.

Intake Guidelines:

For sleep: A range of 3-5 grams of glycine taken orally before bed has been used effectively to help sleep in scientific studies. Bone broth is an excellent source of natural glycine and can contain up to 3 grams of naturally occurring glycine per serving.

Sleep Supporting Hormones

Melatonin

Melatonin is the natural hormone your body releases (endogenous melatonin) that helps to maintain your wake-sleep cycle, also called your biological clock.

Many people are surprised to learn that melatonin is, in fact, a hormone. It's actually the only hormone available in the United States without a prescription because it's considered a dietary supplement. Interestingly, melatonin is regulated, only available with a prescription, and considered a drug in the European Union.

Melatonin (exogenous melatonin) is one of the most used sleep supplements in America. Melatonin is naturally produced both in the brain (pineal gland) as well as in the gut. This popular sleep hormone gets released into the bloodstream as the sun begins to set and is sometimes referenced as the 'Dracula hormone,' the 'hormone of darkness,' and/or the 'vampire hormone.'

Potential challenges with melatonin supplementation: One of the main issues with melatonin supplementation is that it can potentially down-regulate your body's natural ability to utilize melatonin on its own. Remember, melatonin is a hormone, not a vitamin or mineral.

A 2017 study published in the Journal of Clinical Sleep Medicine tested 31 different melatonin supplements bought from grocery stores and pharmacies. Interestingly, scientific evaluation of over-the-counter brands has found melatonin concentrations that range from 83 % less than that claimed on the label to 478 % more than that stated. Also, the amount of melatonin between lots of the same product varied by as much as 465%. This is why I'm not a huge fan of exclusively supplementing with melatonin.

Intake Guidelines:

Effective starting doses to support falling asleep range from 0.3 to 0.5 mg. Bodyweight, health history, metabolism, and the quality and purity of the supplement all factor into dosing.

Lower doses may work great for most people, while others may need a much higher dose, up to 3 mg. Higher doses may be associated with more side effects such as grogginess, headache, and even vivid dreams. Always start with the lowest dose. According to a Cochrane review, doses over 5 mg appear to be no more effective than lower doses.

Vitamin D

Vitamin D is actually a hormone rather than a vitamin. Vitamin D is mostly produced in the skin from sunlight exposure but is also absorbed from a healthy balanced diet. Oily fish such as sardines, mackerel, salmon, oysters, shiitake mushrooms, and egg yolks are good dietary sources of vitamin D. Usually, about 10% of vitamin D is absorbed through eating a healthy diet. About one-half to upwards of three-quarters of U.S. adults are deficient in vitamin D.

Vitamin D levels have been shown to be linked to sleep quality. Vitamin D may help to regulate our circadian clocks. In fact, there is some evidence suggesting that vitamin D may activate two circadian clock genes, which control our 24-hour circadian rhythms.

Intake Guidelines:

A level of 20 nanograms/milliliter to 50 ng/mL is considered adequate for healthy people. A level of less than 12 ng/mL indicates vitamin D deficiency. The best way to know if your vitamin D levels are low is to have your doctor order a blood test. Maintaining sufficient vitamin D levels is good for overall health and wellness, and what's good for your health is also good for your sleep.

Sleep Supporting Vitamins & Minerals

B-Vitamins

Vitamin B6

Vitamin B6 is involved in many functions in the body such as immune health and brain development and function. There's also evidence that B6 aids sleep and can even affect our dreams.

A 2018 study at Australia's University of Adelaide found that vitamin B6 may help people increase their ability to remember their dreams. People with stronger dream recall are more likely to have lucid dream experiences.

A lack of vitamin B6 has been linked to symptoms of insomnia. This could be because vitamin B6 aids in the production of the hormones serotonin and melatonin, both of which are important to sound, restful sleep, and also to mood. Too much vitamin B6, however, is toxic and has been linked to insomnia.

Vitamin B6 is naturally found in bananas, carrots, spinach, potatoes, eggs, cheese, fish, and whole grains.

Vitamin B12

Vitamin B12 is important for brain function and in supporting DNA activity.

Several studies have demonstrated that vitamin B12 is involved in regulating sleep-wake cycles by helping to keep circadian rhythms in sync. That said, the influence of B12 on sleep specifically still isn't very clear. Vitamin B12 is found in eggs, meat, fish, and shellfish.

Intake Guidelines:

The recommended daily allowance (RDA) for adults is 1.3 mg a day of B6. The recommended daily intake (RDI) for vitamin B12 for people over 14 is 2.4 mcg.

Note that the percent of B vitamins that your body can absorb from supplements is usually not very high — it's estimated that your body only absorbs 10 mcg of a 500-mcg B12 supplement.

Minerals

Magnesium - The Master Sleep Mineral

Magnesium is an essential mineral, meaning that our bodies don't produce it, so it must come from outside sources. It's one of seven essential macrominerals that the human body needs in large quantities. We mostly get our magnesium through a healthy diet.

Magnesium deficiency is likely the number one mineral deficiency in the world. Estimates show upwards of 80% of the U.S. population is deficient in magnesium.

Magnesium is responsible for over 300 enzyme reactions and is found in every tissue, but mostly in the brain, bones, and muscles.

In addition, magnesium:

- Plays a key role in energy production, activating ATP, the energy molecule that fuels the body's cells
- Regulates transport of calcium, potassium, and other essential minerals, helping muscles and nerves function properly, and maintaining heart rhythm
- Regulates blood pressure, cholesterol production, and blood glucose levels
- Aids bone development and guards against bone loss
- Functions as an electrolyte, maintaining fluid balance in the body
- Helps control the body's stress-response system and hormones that elevate or diminish stress
- Plays a role in supporting deep, restorative sleep by maintaining healthy levels of GABA, a neurotransmitter that promotes sleep

Research shows that one of the central symptoms of magnesium deficiency is chronic insomnia. People with magnesium deficiency often experience more restless sleep, waking frequently during the night. Research indicates supplemental magnesium can improve sleep quality, especially in people with sleep challenges.

The most effective method of boosting magnesium levels outside of eating more magnesium dense foods (like green leafy veggies, beans, squash, pumpkin and sesame seeds, superfoods like cocoa, spirulina, and brazil nuts) is getting it transdermally -- through a topical application on your skin.

Intake guidelines:

The following doses are based on amounts that have been investigated in scientific studies. In general, it is recommended that users begin with the lowest suggested dose and gradually increase as needed.

For general health, sleep, and stress: 100-420 mg daily. Current U.S. RDA of magnesium for adults is 400 mg – 420 mg/day for men, and 310 mg – 320 mg/day for women. However, often these intake levels (from diet and supplementation combined) are not sufficient to alleviate sleep difficulties. Doubling the intake for a period of time to address the deficiency, and then lowering the dose to maintain a healthy level, is sometimes recommended by functional doctors.

Individual dosing will vary and may vary widely depending on an individual's magnesium levels and the type and quality of the magnesium product. The best forms of oral magnesium supplementation to help with sleep are magnesium glycinate or bisglycinate (glycine increases magnesium absorption and is also calming itself), citrate (also helps with constipation), and orotate. Formulations that contain a mix of all three forms are also highly effective.

Important precaution:

Because of the potential for side effects and interactions with medications, you should only take magnesium or any dietary supplements under the supervision of a knowledgeable health care provider. Some medications may be contraindicated when taking magnesium supplements. Also, people with heart or kidney disease should not take magnesium supplements without supervision. Kidney disorders are known to cause magnesium imbalances, as either too much or too little magnesium is excreted.

Calcium

Calcium is an important sleep-promoting nutrient, as it's necessary for reaching deep sleep cycles and for the brain to produce the sleep-inducing hormone melatonin. Calcium works together with magnesium to relax muscles and is sedating to the nerves; therefore, it's often taken at bedtime to induce sleep.

A study published in the European Neurology Journal identified a link between the absence of deep REM sleep to individuals with calcium deficiencies. Researchers were able to reduce sleep disturbances and normalize sleeping patterns once they restored the blood calcium level of its subjects. This study suggests that calcium supports higher quality and more restful sleep. Calcium may support sleep by helping to convert L-Tryptophan into serotonin and melatonin.

Intake guidelines:

The U.S. RDA for adults is 1,000 mg – 1,300 mg for men and 1,000 mg – 1,300 mg for women. The best and safest sources of calcium come from the foods you eat, like high-quality dairy products such as milk, yogurt, cheese (if tolerated), seeds (sesame seeds are high in calcium), broccoli, kale, salmon, sardines, almonds, legumes, and whole grains.

It's important to note that a balanced ratio of calcium and magnesium in the body is essential to overall health. These two minerals should be taken together in a 2:1 ratio (twice as much calcium as magnesium) for maximum bioavailability.

Zinc

Zinc is the second most abundant trace mineral in the human body after iron. It also happens to be a cofactor in more than 300 enzymes and 1,000 transcription factors that carry out genetic instructions.

Zinc is essential for bone growth, prostate health and male fertility, taste perception, wound healing, and cognitive function. Now researchers find that zinc also may help to regulate sleep, although they are not clear how. In a 2017 study, zinc seemed to promote deep sleep, the kind of sleep we are all seeking more of because of its physical recovery benefits.

Zinc doesn't seem to trigger sleep, but it's been found that adequate levels of zinc in the blood shorten the time it takes to fall asleep (sleep latency), increase the overall amount of sleep, and assure sleep quality and efficiency (time spent asleep when in bed).

The most convincing evidence that zinc consumed in food or supplement is a sleep modulator comes from a Japanese study where mice were fed a yeast extract fortified with either zinc or other minerals. Only the zinc-fed mice experienced a "drastic reduction" in movement at sleep time, and electrical brain recordings showed an increase in the amount of high-quality slow-wave sleep. The researchers believe that once a certain blood level of zinc is reached, it crosses into the brain and activates signaling pathways to promote sleep.

Intake guidelines:

The RDA for zinc is 11 mg/day for males over age 14 and 8 mg/day for females 19 and older. Natural foods with high levels of zinc include oysters, grass-fed meat, and wheat germ.

If you are looking to get more sleep-promoting vitamins, amino acids, and minerals naturally from your diet, here is a chart to help you:

Supplement	Helps With	Also Found In
Vitamin B	Regulation of tryptophan Produces serotonin	Chicken breast Lean beef Salmon Bananas Potatoes
Vitamin D	Helps regulate circadian rhythms	Sardines Mackerel Salmon Oysters Shiitake mushrooms Egg yolks
Calcium	Relaxant	Dark leafy greens Cruciferous vegetables High-quality dairy
Zinc	Deficiency is linked to insomnia	Oysters Grass-fed beef
Magnesium	Helps to relax the body Deficiency is linked to insomnia	Avocado Nuts Legumes Tofu
Glycine	Lowers body temperature, signaling time for sleep	Bone broth Grass-fed meat Eggs, kale, spinach
Gaba	Lower anxiety Creates a calm mood	Green, black, and oolong tea Kefir and yogurt Tempeh
L-theanine	Promotes relaxation Increases focus and creativity	Green tea

PART 4

Conclusion

Sleep Troubleshooting

What do you do when you've tried all the environmental and new bed-time rituals and still have issues sleeping? Frequently those who suffer from insomnia will try to force themselves to sleep. This type of mental energy only compounds the problem. From my experience, the closest thing to a silver bullet for sleep is releasing expectations and attempting to force or will yourself to sleep.

I've found this simple sleep mindset shift to be very helpful for the high achievers that I personally work with who continue to have sleep challenges despite implementing all the new rituals and environmental changes.

Most of us are always looking for ways to improve and achieve more. This is a baseline human drive. Although this mindset in most cases is extremely helpful and often leads to success, when it comes to getting deep, restorative, restful sleep, it's actually the one thing that may prevent us from getting more of it.

Releasing expectations and the will to sleep means fully accepting the current reality. Accepting reality by choosing to experience it versus resisting it, making it wrong, or worrying about it. Releasing expectations allows any mental, emotional, or physical tension, stress, or resistance to be surrendered and, more often than not, leads to sleep.

Sometimes, it's by simply letting go of trying to control things that allows us to relax into what we truly desire; in this case, restful sleep. This is because attempting to force yourself to sleep can and will create more frustration and stress, and it's that frustration and stress that keeps you awake. It truly is a paradox.

Have you ever heard the saying, *What you resist, persists?* When it comes to getting and staying asleep, this little phrase holds very true. **Resisting not being able to sleep, persists not being able to sleep.** Acceptance allows us to experience the desired result; in this case, sleep. Sleep is something that cannot be forced, and trying to do so is a losing sleep battle.

So how does one actually accomplish this? It begins with accepting the current condition by acknowledging how you feel. After checking in with how you feel, whether it's anxious, frustrated, stressed, etc., the next step is to simply take 12 deep breaths into your diaphragm (stomach) while repeating either in your mind or out loud and softly, the word 'release.'

Then begin to notice the thoughts that appear in your mind while you're breathing. Are these thoughts stress-inducing or sleep-inducing? An example of a stress-inducing thought is that if *I don't get to sleep in the next five minutes, my day will be wrecked tomorrow.* An example of a sleep-inducing thought would be, *how lucky am I to have a comfortable, warm bed to sleep in.* This sleep practice takes practice, and it may take a few rounds of 'releasing' before you'll begin to notice the negative feelings soon pass and you fall into a deep peaceful sleep.[6]

Do You Have Sleep Apnea?

Sleep apnea is the second-largest sleep disorder outside of insomnia. It is estimated that 22 million Americans suffer from sleep apnea, with 85% of the cases of moderate and severe obstructive sleep apnea undiagnosed. This means that many people suffer from sleep apnea and don't even know it. Sleep apnea disrupts more than just your good night's sleep. It's a risk factor for heart attack, stroke, diabetes, and other serious health conditions.

But what is sleep apnea? Sleep apnea is a sleep disorder in which breathing repeatedly stops and starts. This happens when you lie down to sleep and the muscles in your throat relax. This may lead to a shift in the tongue or soft palate, causing your airway to narrow so much that it briefly closes off completely. A disruption in your breathing can then reduce the level of oxygen in the blood. Drops in oxygen levels alert your brain that something isn't working as it should. As a result, the brain wakes the sleeping person up so the airway can be reopened. This becomes a problem when the sleeping person is woken up over and over again, sometimes dozens of times an hour. Repeated awakenings lead to a deficit in deep, restorative sleep.

There are three main types of sleep apnea:

- Obstructive sleep apnea, the more common form that occurs when throat muscles relax

---

[6] This is just one of the mind-body techniques we teach our clients at Sleep Science Academy. If you need more support with your sleep, helping people get and stay asleep is what we do. Visit www.SleepScienceAcademy.com

- Central sleep apnea, which occurs when your brain doesn't send proper signals to the muscles that control breathing
- Complex sleep apnea syndrome, also known as treatment-emergent central sleep apnea, when someone has both obstructive sleep apnea and central sleep apnea

How do you know if you have sleep apnea?

If you snore loudly and feel tired even after a full night's sleep, you might have sleep apnea. A number of risk factors can increase the likelihood of sleep apnea, such as being overweight or obese, having a large neck circumference (more than 17" in men and more than 16" in women), genetically passed-down characteristics such as a naturally narrow airway, consuming alcohol close to bedtime, and smoking. Although it is statistically more common for an older, overweight man to have sleep apnea symptoms, sleep apnea can affect anyone: children, women, and even athletes. If you suspect you have sleep apnea, start by downloading the Sleep Cycle app and recording yourself through the night. Snoring is a sign you may have sleep apnea. Then ask your doctor about having an overnight sleep study. Such studies are the most accurate way to diagnose sleep apnea. If you don't have insurance or desire to sleep in a sleep lab, there is also a pretty precise sleep apnea home device called the SleepTuner™, which is a little device you wear on your forehead for a few nights. The SleepTuner™ was engineered to measure and assess stopped breathing events, and takes the science found in a sleep lab and puts it into a device small enough to fit in your pocket. It monitors heart rate, sleep position, breathing, and more with clinical-grade accuracy, then generates reports that are easy to understand and act on. [7]

There are ways to deal with sleep apnea. Weight loss can help and does, in most cases, especially if you are very overweight. In one of my seminars, a participant shared this story:

---

[7] Learn more at https://www.beddrsleep.com

I had high blood pressure, was diagnosed with sleep apnea, and felt terrible all the time. My diet was crap, and I wasn't exercising. I didn't want to wear the CPAP, and my wife looked at me and said, 'why don't you try changing your diet and losing the beer gut!' The truth was, she was right, so I did, and eight weeks later, after changing my diet and exercising, I lost 20 lbs and didn't need the blood pressure medication or the CPAP machine anymore.

Avoiding alcohol and sleeping on your back can also make a difference. During a study on the significance of body posture on breathing abnormalities during sleep, 574 patients with sleep apnea had at least double as many instances of apneas/hypopnea when sleeping on their back as compared to sleeping on their side. But for some, even these simple changes won't work, which is why PAP (positive airway pressure) therapy - a mask that promotes airflow during sleep - is usually the recommended treatment. If your doctor diagnoses sleep apnea and prescribes PAP therapy, be prepared to commit to the treatment. If you want to try something a little esoteric, you could try mouth taping and using a Breathe Right strip. By unblocking the nose and switching to nasal breathing during the night, you reduce breathing volume and snoring, and sleep apnea can be significantly reduced. There is a company called Sommex that sells tape specifically designed for this purpose![8]

---

[8] You can learn more about the benefits of nighttime nasal breathing by visiting https://buteykoclinic.com/sleepapnea

Now Decide

Everything begins with a decision. **Experiencing how extraordinary our body and mind are designed to feel doesn't happen by chance. It happens by choice.** Life is full of choices and the little choices we decide to make and not make shape our health, life, and destiny.

The quality of our lives comes down to the quality of our decisions. Making a consistent decision to prioritize and protect our sleep helps us make better decisions, thus compounding the improvement of our lives. The decision to intentionally improve sleep is life-changing. Think about the choices you've made in the past and how those choices massively impacted your life.

In order to create and feel sustained natural energy consistently throughout life, we must fully commit to a higher standard of health. It's this commitment that supports us to protect our greatest asset, our health. Sleep is the foundation of extraordinary health. It keeps our bodies healthy and our minds clear. It reduces our chances of disease drastically. It can make us smarter, more confident, and more productive. It releases stress and tension from our bodies and brings peace to our minds.

Leverage these facts to fuel your commitment to protect and prioritize sleep. Who needs you to show up now? Who needs you to be more committed to your energy, health, and performance? Is it your spouse? Kids? Employees or co-workers? Community? Church? Mission?

Study after study has shown that increasing the quality of sleep does increase our daytime energy and our ability to focus and boost our mood.

After realizing that sleep is the foundation on which extraordinary health is built and how much quality sleep impacts productivity and performance, I decided to test the ROI of excellent sleep for myself.[9] So, I took 20 high performers between the ages of 25-65 and ran them through a 6-week sleep and performance case study program to measure how sleep quality impacted daytime energy levels, cognitive performance, and emotional health. Our constants in the study were a consistent bed and rise time (a foundation for quality sleep), eliminating alcohol (a known disturber of quality sleep), and limiting caffeine after 12 pm (also a known sleep quality disruptor). Then each week, we tested one of the following sleep variables.

The first week we tested a 10-minute meditation to see how reducing stress before bed affects sleep quality. In the second week, we tested a 90-minute screen curfew to eliminate blue-light exposure. The third week we tested a 3-hour fasting window - which means no food three hours before bed. In the fourth week, we tested creating an optimal sleep environment: cold (65 degrees), dark, and quiet. In the fifth week, we tested taking 'energy breaks' about 10 minutes in length each hour to recover from stress throughout the workday. In the last week, we tested a doctor-formulated sleep supplement designed to help overcome the most common nutritional deficiencies that can interfere with deep, restorative sleep.

Here are the results and conclusions of the study:

90% of the participants reported feeling more energy and focus, and were happier during the weeks they got higher quality sleep. This was not a huge surprise. It was surprising that there was no one-size-fits-all sleep experiment that increased sleep quality across all the participants. Specific sleep experiments increased sleep quality for certain people, and others did not. When it comes to increasing sleep quality, it's not a one-size-fits-all solution. I believe sleep is as individual as diet and exercise. Prioritizing

---

[9]   To learn more about the sleep and performance case study, watch my TEDx talk titled "The ROI of Sleep" on YouTube.

sleep can help us better prepare for when 'life happens.' During the six-week study, certain participants had life events that affected the quality of their sleep. For example, one participant had to undergo surgery, another traveled across several time zones, and another sacrificed his sleep for a couple of days to support a family member during a difficult time. Interestingly, but not surprisingly, these life events all showed up in the quality of their sleep. The participants reported that by making their sleep a priority, they could handle these stressful life events better. Sleep can truly help us be better prepared when 'life happens.'

The way to capitalize on the ROI of great sleep is first and foremost through prioritizing and protecting it. Unfortunately, sleep is usually the first thing that gets put on the back burner when the *shit hits the fan*. By making a new decision to create a nonnegotiable 8-hour sleep window or sleep opportunity each night and giving yourself permission to rest, recharge, and reset, you'll be better prepared for life. Despite how it may feel sometimes, life isn't an emergency! We truly have more control over our lives than we realize.

The second way to capitalize on the ROI of great sleep is by measuring it. We manage what we measure, and we now have many fantastic tools to track sleep quantity and quality accurately. The device we used in the sleep study tracks carefully essential sleep data; for example, time in bed asleep, how fast you fall asleep, body temperature, resting heart rate, and heart rate variability, as well as the different sleep stages. Measuring sleep provides the necessary feedback we need to continue to experiment with our sleep. If you think about it, life is just one big experiment. We try something and we get feedback; we try something else and we get feedback. While experimenting, avoid the trap of getting caught up in all the complex health dogma and obsessing over it.

The third way to capitalize on the ROI of great sleep is by learning to master stress. Stress and sleep are so closely connected. The interconnected bi-directional relationship between sleep and stress can't be under-estimated. Learning to be better at stress is the key to improving sleep and vice versa.

It's the small, consistent things that we do every day, those little choices we make, that determine if we'll experience how good our bodies are designed to feel.

As we choose to create and live our healthiest best selves, we give others permission to do the same—sustained, natural, vibrant energy ripples out into families, friends, communities, and companies. Sleep is the first step to restoring our energy edge, which is contagious and magnetic. When those you live with and those you lead see you ascending to a higher level of energy and health, it will inspire them to take new elevated action creating a positive ripple effect. Now more than ever we need more good people to step up and demonstrate what's possible and to lead others by example. As Gandhi so wisely shared, *be the change you want to see in others.*

If you've made it this far, you've likely already started taking some new elevated action and are sleeping better because of it, and I want to acknowledge you for that. If you found the information in this book valuable, please share it with those you care most about.

Sleep truly is one of the best ways we can spend our time to protect our health, our sanity, and to accelerate our overall performance. Sleep is the secret to success and the ROI of sleep is worth the nightly invest-ment because getting quality sleep improves every aspect of our lives - our health, relationships, careers, and performance.

I hope from reading this book that you no longer sacrifice sleep, no lon-ger see it as a luxury or as wasted time, and that you rethink the all too common phrase...*when you snooze, you lose.* Because now you know, *when you snooze, you win!*...sweet dreams.

To continue your sleep and performance journey, please visit www.SleepScienceAcademy.com to learn more about how we can support you. We offer programs using the most cutting edge, unique, and holistic approaches, all based in science, that have helped hundreds of clients get and stay asleep all night long. Our mission at Sleep Science Academy is to give people the tools and support they need to stop suffering and start sleeping as soon as possible. We help our clients get and stay asleep each night, even if they've "tried everything" and have been struggling for years.

References

PREFACE

Kripke, D., Langer, R., Kline, L. (2012). Hypnotics' association with mortality or cancer: a matched cohort study. BMJ Open 2, no.1: e00850.

PART 1: SLEEP THE MISSING LINK

Beccuti, Guglielmo, and Silvana Pannain. "Sleep and Obesity." Current Opinion in Clinical Nutrition and Metabolic Care, U.S. National Library of Medicine, July 2011, www.ncbi.nlm.nih.gov/pmc/articles/PMC3632337/.

Dimitrov, Stoyan, and Tanja Lange. "G Protein-Coupled Receptor Signaling." Journal of Experimental Medicine, 12 Feb. 2019, doi: 10.32388/g4au30.

Nedeltcheva, A., et al. (2010). Insufficient Sleep Undermines Dietary Efforts to Reduce Adiposity. Annals of Internal Medicine, U.S. National Library of Medicine, 5 Oct. 2010, www.ncbi.nlm.nih.gov/pmc/articles/PMC2951287.

Walker, M. (2018). Why We Sleep: Unlocking the Power of Sleep and Dreams. Scribner, an Imprint of Simon and Schuster, Inc.

PART 2: MASTERING SLEEP

Amutio, Alberto, et al. "Effects of Mindfulness Training on Sleep Problems in Patients With Fibromyalgia." Frontiers, Frontiers, 16 July 2018, www.frontiersin.org/articles/10.3389/fpsyg.2018.01365/full.

Breus, M. (2019). The Power of When: Discover Your Chronotype--and Learn the Best Time to Eat Lunch, Ask for a Raise, Have Sex, Write a Novel, Take Your Meds, and More. Little, Brown Spark.

Black, David S, et al. "Mindfulness Meditation and Improvement in Sleep Quality and Daytime Impairment among Older Adults with Sleep Disturbances: a Randomized Clinical Trial." JAMA Internal Medicine, U.S. National Library of Medicine, Apr. 2015, www.ncbi.nlm.nih.gov/pmc/articles/PMC4407465/ www.health.harvard.edu/blog/mindfulness-meditation-helps-fight-insomnia-improves-sleep-201502187726.

Garman, Susan Sorenson and Keri, and Keri Garman. "How to Tackle U.S. Employees' Stagnating Engagement." Gallup.com, Gallup, 11 June 2013, news.gallup.com/businessjournal/162953/tackle-employees-stagnating-engagement.aspx?g_source=link_newsv9.

Gordon, Amie M., and Serena Chen. "The Role of Sleep in Interpersonal Conflict." Social Psychological and Personality Science, vol. 5, no. 2, 2013, pp. 168–175., doi:10.1177/1948550613488952.

Northwestern University. (2017, July 10). Purpose in life by day linked to better sleep at night: Older adults whose lives have meaning enjoy better sleep quality, less sleep apnea, restless leg syndrome. ScienceDaily. Retrieved July 21, 2020 from www.sciencedaily.com/releases/2017/07/170710091734.htm

"Poor Sleep Is Associated with Lower Relationship Satisfaction in Both Women and Men." *American Academy of Sleep Medicine – Association for Sleep Clinicians and Researchers*, 2 June 2009, aasm.org/poor-sleep-is-associated-with-lower-relationship-satisfaction-in-both-women-and-men/.

Richter, K. et al. (2016). Two in a Bed: The Influence of Couple Sleeping and Chronotypes on Relationship and Sleep. An Overview. Chronobiology International, Taylor & Francis. www.ncbi.nlm.nih.gov/pmc/articles/PMC5152533/.

Rodriguez, Tori. "Laugh Lots, Live Longer." Scientific American, Scientific American, 1 Sept. 2016, www.scientificamerican.com/article/laugh-lots-live-longer/.

Turner, Arlener. "Purpose in Life by Day Linked to Better Sleep at Night." EurekAlert!, 9 July 2017, www.eurekalert.org/pub_releases/2017-07/nu-pil070617.php.

PART 3: SUPPORTING SLEEP

Abbasi, B. et al. (2012). The Effect of Magnesium Supplementation on Primary Insomnia in Elderly: A Double-Blind Placebo-Controlled Clinical Trial. *Journal of Research in Medical Sciences: the Official Journal of Isfahan University of Medical Sciences*, Medknow Publications & Media Pvt Ltd, Dec. 2012, www.ncbi.nlm.nih.gov/pubmed/23853635.

Bannai, Makoto, et al. "Oral Administration of Glycine Increases Extracellular Serotonin but Not Dopamine in the Prefrontal Cortex of Rats." *Psychiatry and Clinical Neurosciences*, U.S. National Library of Medicine, Mar. 2011, www.ncbi.nlm.nih.gov/pubmed/21414089.

Bertisch, Suzanne M, et al. "25-Hydroxyvitamin D Concentration and Sleep Duration and Continuity: Multi-Ethnic Study of Atherosclerosis." *Sleep*, Associated Professional Sleep Societies, LLC, 1 Aug. 2015, www.ncbi.nlm.nih.gov/pmc/articles/PMC4507736/.

Boonstra, Evert, et al. "Neurotransmitters as Food Supplements: the Effects of GABA on Brain and Behavior." *Frontiers in Psychology*, Frontiers Media S.A., 6 Oct. 2015, www.ncbi.nlm.nih.gov/pmc/articles/PMC4594160/.

Booz, George W. "Cannabidiol as an Emergent Therapeutic Strategy for Lessening the Impact of Inflammation on Oxidative Stress." *Free Radical Biology & Medicine*, U.S. National Library of Medicine, 1 Sept. 2011, www.ncbi.nlm.nih.gov/pubmed/21238581.

Breus, Michael. "Understanding L-Theanine: Sleep Better at Night, Feel Relaxed and Alert during the Day." *Your Guide to Better Sleep*, 31 May 2018, www.thesleepdoctor.com/2017/07/11/understanding-l-theanine-sleep-better-night-feel-relaxed-alert-day/.

Breus, Michael. "Understanding L-Theanine: Sleep Better at Night, Feel Relaxed and Alert during the Day." *Your Guide to Better Sleep*, 31 May 2018, www.thesleepdoctor.com/2017/07/11/understanding-l-theanine-sleep-better-night-feel-relaxed-alert-day/.

Breus, Michael. "Understanding Valerian and Hops." *Your Guide to Better Sleep*, 30 Jan. 2018, www.thesleepdoctor.com/2017/06/19/understanding-valerian-hops-how-valerian-and-hops-can-help-you-de-stress-relax-and-sleep-better/.

Breus, Michael. "5 Vitamin Deficiencies That Can Affect Your Sleep." *Your Guide to Better Sleep*, 13 Feb. 2019, www.thesleepdoctor.com/2019/02/12/5-vitamin-deficiencies-that-can-affect-your-sleep/.

Breus, Michael. "5 Vitamin Deficiencies That Can Affect Your Sleep." *Your Guide to Better Sleep*, 13 Feb. 2019, www.thesleepdoctor. com/2019/02/12/5-vitamin-deficiencies-that-can-affect-your-sleep/.

Breus, Michael. "The Connection Between Glycine and Sleep." *Your Guide to Better Sleep*, 24 July 2018, www.thesleepdoctor.com/2018/07/23/ understanding-glycine/.

Breus, Micheal. "Understanding CBD: The Calming and Sleep Promoting Benefits of Cannabidiol." *Your Guide to Better Sleep*, 12 Aug. 2019, www.thesleepdoctor.com/2017/08/10/understanding-cbd/.

Brues. Micheal. "Magnesium - How It Affects Your Sleep." *Your Guide to Better Sleep*, 27 Oct. 2019, www.thesleepdoctor.com/2017/11/20/ magnesium-effects-sleep/.

Butterweck, Veronika, et al. "Hypothermic Effects of Hops Are Antagonized with the Competitive Melatonin Receptor Antagonist Luzindole in Mice." *The Journal of Pharmacy and Pharmacology*, U.S. National Library of Medicine, Apr. 2007, www.ncbi.nlm.nih.gov/ pubmed/17430638.

Carmel, Ralph. "How I Treat Cobalamin (Vitamin B12) Deficiency." *Blood*, American Society of Hematology, 15 Sept. 2008, www.ncbi.nlm. nih.gov/pubmed/18606874.

Cases, Julien, et al. "Pilot Trial of Melissa Officinalis L. Leaf Extract in the Treatment of Volunteers Suffering from Mild-to-Moderate Anxiety Disorders and Sleep Disturbances." *Mediterranean Journal of Nutrition and Metabolism*, Springer Milan, Dec. 2011, www.ncbi.nlm.nih.gov/ pmc/articles/PMC3230760/.

CBS News. (2015). Herbal Supplements Filled with Fake Ingredients, Investigators Find. CBS News, CBS Interactive, Feb. 2015, www.cbsnews. com/news/herbal-supplements-targeted-by-new-york-attorney-general/

Chagas, Marcos Hortes N, et al. "Effects of Acute Systemic Administration of Cannabidiol on Sleep-Wake Cycle in Rats - Marcos Hortes N Chagas, José Alexandre S Crippa, Antonio Waldo Zuardi, Jaime E C Hallak, João Paulo Machado-De-Sousa, Camila Hirotsu, Lucas Maia, Sergio Tufik, Monica Levy Andersen, 2013." *SAGE Journals*, www.journals.sagepub. com/doi/abs/10.1177/0269881112474524.

Cherasse, Yoan, and Yoshihiro Urade. "Dietary Zinc Acts as a Sleep Modulator." *International Journal of Molecular Sciences*, MDPI, 5 Nov. 2017, www.ncbi.nlm.nih.gov/pmc/articles/PMC5713303/.

Cohen, Pieter A, et al. "Prohibited Stimulants in Dietary Supplements After Enforcement Action by the US Food and Drug Administration." JAMA Internal Medicine, American Medical Association, 1 Dec. 2018, www.ncbi.nlm.nih.gov/pmc/articles/PMC6583602/.

Costello, Rebecca B, et al. "The Effectiveness of Melatonin for Promoting Healthy Sleep: A Rapid Evidence Assessment of the Literature." *Nutrition Journal*, BioMed Central, 7 Nov. 2014, www.ncbi.nlm.nih.gov/pmc/articles/PMC4273450/.

Crighton, Elly, et al. "Toxicological Screening and DNA Sequencing Detects Contamination and Adulteration in Regulated Herbal Medicines and Supplements for Diet, Weight Loss and Cardiovascular Health." Journal of Pharmaceutical and Biomedical Analysis, U.S. National Library of Medicine, 30 Nov. 2019, www.ncbi.nlm.nih.gov/pubmed/31472365.

Cunha, J M, et al. "Chronic Administration of Cannabidiol to Healthy Volunteers and Epileptic Patients." *Pharmacology*, U.S.

National Library of Medicine, 1980, www.ncbi.nlm.nih.gov/pubmed/7413719?dopt=Abstract.

Donath, F, et al. "Critical Evaluation of the Effect of Valerian Extract on Sleep Structure and Sleep Quality." *Pharmacopsychiatry*, U.S. National Library of Medicine, Mar. 2000, www.ncbi.nlm.nih.gov/pubmed/10761819.

Drugs.com. Melatonin: Side Effects, Uses, Dosage (Kids/Adults). *Drugs.com*, www.drugs.com/melatonin.html.

Elikkottil, Jaseena, et al. "The Analgesic Potential of Cannabinoids." *Journal of Opioid Management*, U.S. National Library of Medicine, 2009, www.ncbi.nlm.nih.gov/pmc/articles/PMC3728280/.

Emanuele, Enzo, et al. "An Open-Label Trial of L-5-Hydroxytryptophan in Subjects with Romantic Stress." *Neuroendocrinology Letters*, U.S. National Library of Medicine, 2010, www.ncbi.nlm.nih.gov/pubmed/21178946.

Franco, L, et al. "The Sedative Effects of Hops (Humulus Lupulus), a Component of Beer, on the Activity/Rest Rhythm." *Acta Physiologica Hungarica*, U.S. National Library of Medicine, June 2012, www.ncbi.nlm.nih.gov/pubmed/22849837.

Gao, Qi, et al. "The Association between Vitamin D Deficiency and Sleep Disorders: A Systematic Review and Meta-Analysis." Nutrients, MDPI, 1 Oct. 2018, www.ncbi.nlm.nih.gov/pmc/articles/PMC6213953/.

Grandner, Michael A, et al. "Sleep Symptoms Associated with Intake of Specific Dietary Nutrients." *Journal of Sleep Research*, U.S. National Library of Medicine, Feb. 2014, www.ncbi.nlm.nih.gov/pmc/articles/PMC3866235/.

Grandner, Michael A, et al. "Sleep Symptoms Associated with Intake of Specific Dietary Nutrients." *Journal of Sleep Research*, U.S. National Library of Medicine, Feb. 2014, www.ncbi.nlm.nih.gov/pmc/articles/PMC3866235/.

Grigg-Damberger, Madeleine M, and Dessislava Ianakieva. "Poor Quality Control of Over-the-Counter Melatonin: What They Say Is Often Not What You Get." *Journal of Clinical Sleep Medicine : JCSM : Official Publication of the American Academy of Sleep Medicine*, American Academy of Sleep Medicine, 15 Feb. 2017, www.ncbi.nlm.nih.gov/pmc/articles/PMC5263069/.

Hampson, A J, et al. "Cannabidiol and (-)Delta9-Tetrahydrocannabinol Are Neuroprotective Antioxidants." *Proceedings of the National Academy of Sciences of the United States of America*, National Academy of Sciences, 7 July 1998, www.ncbi.nlm.nih.gov/pmc/articles/PMC20965/.

Han, Bin, et al. "Association between Serum Vitamin D Levels and Sleep Disturbance in Hemodialysis Patients." *Nutrients*, MDPI, 14 Feb. 2017, www.ncbi.nlm.nih.gov/pmc/articles/PMC5331570/.

Harvard Health Publishing. "Getting Enough Vitamin B12." *Harvard Health*, www.health.harvard.edu/vitamins-and-supplements/getting-enough-vitamin-b12.

Held, Katja, et al. "Oral Mg(2+) Supplementation Reverses Age-Related Neuroendocrine and Sleep EEG Changes in Humans." *Pharmacopsychiatry*, U.S. National Library of Medicine, July 2002, www.ncbi.nlm.nih.gov/pubmed/12163983.

HJ; Hong KB; Park Y; Suh. "Sleep-Promoting Effects of a GABA/5-HTP Mixture: Behavioral Changes and Neuromodulation in an Invertebrate

Model." *Life Sciences*, U.S. National Library of Medicine, pubmed.ncbi. nlm.nih.gov/26921634/.

Hong, Ki-Bae, et al. "Sleep-Promoting Effects of the GABA/5-HTP Mixture in Vertebrate Models." *Behavioural Brain Research*, U.S. National Library of Medicine, 1 Sept. 2016, www.ncbi.nlm.nih.gov/ pubmed/27150227.

Jung, Young Saeng, et al. "The Relationship between Serum Vitamin D Levels and Sleep Quality in Fixed Day Indoor Field Workers in the Electronics Manufacturing Industry in Korea." *Annals of Occupational and Environmental Medicine*, BioMed Central, 24 June 2017, www.ncbi. nlm.nih.gov/pubmed/28652922.

Karabin, Marcel, et al. "Biotransformations and Biological Activities of Hop Flavonoids." *Biotechnology Advances*, U.S. National Library of Medicine, 1 Nov. 2015, www.ncbi.nlm.nih.gov/pubmed/25708386.

Kawai, Nobuhiro, et al. "The Sleep-Promoting and Hypothermic Effects of Glycine Are Mediated by NMDA Receptors in the Suprachiasmatic Nucleus." *Neuropsychopharmacology : Official Publication of the American College of Neuropsychopharmacology*, Nature Publishing Group, May 2015, www.ncbi.nlm.nih.gov/pubmed/25533534.

Kawai, Nobuhiro, et al. "The Sleep-Promoting and Hypothermic Effects of Glycine Are Mediated by NMDA Receptors in the Suprachiasmatic Nucleus." *Neuropsychopharmacology : Official Publication of the American College of Neuropsychopharmacology*, Nature Publishing Group, May 2015, www.ncbi.nlm.nih.gov/pubmed/25533534.

Kennedy, David O, et al. "Attenuation of Laboratory-Induced Stress in Humans after Acute Administration of Melissa Officinalis (Lemon

Balm)." *Psychosomatic Medicine*, U.S. National Library of Medicine, 2004, www.ncbi.nlm.nih.gov/pubmed/15272110.

Kimura, Kenta, et al. "L-Theanine Reduces Psychological and Physiological Stress Responses." *Biological Psychology*, U.S. National Library of Medicine, Jan. 2007, www.ncbi.nlm.nih.gov/pubmed/16930802.

Leathwood, P D, et al. "Aqueous Extract of Valerian Root (Valeriana Officinalis L.) Improves Sleep Quality in Man." *Pharmacology, Biochemistry, and Behavior*, U.S. National Library of Medicine, July 1982, www.ncbi.nlm.nih.gov/pubmed/7122669.

Lindahl, O, and L Lindwall. "Double-Blind Study of a Valerian Preparation." *Pharmacology, Biochemistry, and Behavior*, U.S. National Library of Medicine, Apr. 1989, www.ncbi.nlm.nih.gov/pubmed/2678162.

Linus Pauling Institute. (2020). Vitamin B6. 1 Jan. 2020, lpi.oregonstate.edu/mic/vitamins/vitamin-B6.

Lite, Jordan. "Vitamin D Deficiency Soars in the U.S., Study Says." *Scientific American*, Scientific American, 23 Mar. 2009, www.scientificamerican.com/article/vitamin-d-deficiency-united-states/.

L.A. Erland and P.K Saxena, "Melatonin natural health products and supplements; presence of serotonin and significant variability of melatonin content," Journal of Clinical Sleep Medicine 2017;13(2);275-81

Mackie, K. "Cannabinoid Receptors: Where They Are and What They Do." *Journal of Neuroendocrinology*, U.S. National Library of Medicine, May 2008, www.ncbi.nlm.nih.gov/pubmed/18426493.

Malhotra, Samir, et al. "The Therapeutic Potential of Melatonin: a Review of the Science." *MedGenMed : Medscape General Medicine*, Medscape, 13 Apr. 2004, www.ncbi.nlm.nih.gov/pmc/articles/PMC1395802/.

Marano, Hara Estroff. "Zzzz-Zinc." *Psychology Today*, Sussex Publishers, 2 July 2018, www.psychologytoday.com/us/articles/201807/zzzz-zinc.

Melatonin for the Prevention and Treatment of Jet Lag, www.cochrane.org/CD001520/DEPRESSN_melatonin-for-the-prevention-and-treatment-of-jet-lag.

Meyerhoff, Dieter J, et al. "Cortical Gamma-Aminobutyric Acid and Glutamate in Posttraumatic Stress Disorder and Their Relationships to Self-Reported Sleep Quality." *Sleep*, Associated Professional Sleep Societies, LLC, 1 May 2014, www.ncbi.nlm.nih.gov/pubmed/24790267.

Meyerhoff, Dieter J, et al. "Cortical Gamma-Aminobutyric Acid and Glutamate in Posttraumatic Stress Disorder and Their Relationships to Self-Reported Sleep Quality." *Sleep*, Associated Professional Sleep Societies, LLC, 1 May 2014, www.ncbi.nlm.nih.gov/pubmed/24790267.

Miranda, C L, et al. "Antiproliferative and Cytotoxic Effects of Prenylated Flavonoids from Hops (Humulus Lupulus) in Human Cancer Cell Lines." *Food and Chemical Toxicology: An International Journal Published for the British Industrial Biological Research Association*, U.S. National Library of Medicine, Apr. 1999, www.ncbi.nlm.nih.gov/pubmed/10418944.

Morin, Charles M, et al. "Valerian-Hops Combination and Diphenhydramine for Treating Insomnia: a Randomized Placebo-Controlled Clinical Trial." *Sleep*, U.S. National Library of Medicine, Nov. 2005, www.ncbi.nlm.nih.gov/pubmed/16335333.

Möykkynen, T, et al. "Magnesium Potentiation of the Function of Native and Recombinant GABA(A) Receptors." *Neuroreport*, U.S. National Library of Medicine, 20 July 2001, www.ncbi.nlm.nih.gov/pubmed/11447329.

Naima, et al. "Top 2 Sleep Promoting Nutrients: Magnesium and Calcium." *Naturimedica*, 31 July 2019, www.naturimedica.com/top-2-sleep-promoting-nutrients-magnesium-and-calcium/.

Naima, et al. "Top 2 Sleep Promoting Nutrients: Magnesium and Calcium." *Naturimedica*, 31 July 2019, www.naturimedica.com/top-2-sleep-promoting-nutrients-magnesium-and-calcium/.

Nielsen, Forrest H, et al. "Magnesium Supplementation Improves Indicators of Low Magnesium Status and Inflammatory Stress in Adults Older than 51 Years with Poor Quality Sleep." *Magnesium Research*, U.S. National Library of Medicine, Dec. 2010, www.ncbi.nlm.nih.gov/pubmed/21199787.

Pyndt Jørgensen, Bettina, et al. "Dietary Magnesium Deficiency Affects Gut Microbiota and Anxiety-like Behaviour in C57BL/6N Mice." *Acta Neuropsychiatrica*, U.S. National Library of Medicine, Oct. 2015, www.ncbi.nlm.nih.gov/pubmed/25773775.

Savage, Crispin. "Want to Remember Your Dreams? Try Taking Vitamin B6." *Medical Xpress - Medical Research Advances and Health News*, Medical Xpress, 27 Apr. 2018, medicalxpress.com/news/2018-04-vitamin-b6.html.

ScienceDaily. (2015). Calcium Channel Essential for Deep Sleep Identified. *ScienceDaily*, 27 June 2015, www.sciencedaily.com/releases/2015/06/150627081214.htm.

Stańska, Katarzyna, and Antonii Krzeski. "The Umami Taste: from Discovery to Clinical Use." *Otolaryngologia Polska = The Polish Otolaryngology*, U.S. National Library of Medicine, 30 June 2016, www. ncbi.nlm.nih.gov/pubmed/27387211.

Suhner, A, et al. "Comparative Study to Determine the Optimal Melatonin Dosage Form for the Alleviation of Jet Lag." *Chronobiology International*, U.S. National Library of Medicine, Nov. 1998, www.ncbi. nlm.nih.gov/pubmed/9844753.

Taavoni, S, et al. "Valerian/Lemon Balm Use for Sleep Disorders during Menopause." *Complementary Therapies in Clinical Practice*, U.S. National Library of Medicine, Nov. 2013, www.ncbi.nlm.nih.gov/ pubmed/24199972.

Taavoni, Simin, et al. "Effect of Valerian on Sleep Quality in Postmenopausal Women: a Randomized Placebo-Controlled Clinical Trial." *Menopause (New York, N.Y.)*, U.S. National Library of Medicine, Sept. 2011, www.ncbi.nlm.nih.gov/pubmed/21775910.

U.S. Department of Health and Human Services. Office of Dietary Supplements - Vitamin B6."\ *NIH Office of Dietary Supplements*, ods. od.nih.gov/factsheets/VitaminB6-HealthProfessional/.

Vural, Esmée M S, et al. "Optimal Dosages for Melatonin Supplementation Therapy in Older Adults: a Systematic Review of Current Literature." *Drugs & Aging*, U.S. National Library of Medicine, June 2014, www. ncbi.nlm.nih.gov/pubmed/24802882.

Winkelman, John W, et al. "Reduced Brain GABA in Primary Insomnia: Preliminary Data from 4T Proton Magnetic Resonance Spectroscopy (1H-MRS)." Sleep, Associated Professional Sleep Societies, LLC, Nov. 2008, www.ncbi.nlm.nih.gov/pmc/articles/PMC2579978/.

116 | THE SLEEP ADVANTAGE

Yamadera, Wataru, et al. "Glycine Ingestion Improves Subjective Sleep Quality in Human Volunteers, Correlating with Polysomnographic Changes." *Wiley Online Library*, John Wiley & Sons, Ltd, 27 Mar. 2007, onlinelibrary.wiley.com/doi/full/10.1111/j.1479-8425.2007.00262.x.

Zadeh, et al. "Comparison of Nutrient Intake by Sleep Status in Selected Adults in Mysore, India." *Https://Doi.org/10.4162/Nrp.2011.5.3.230*, synapse.koreamed.org/search.php?where=aview&id=10.4162%2Fnrp.2011.5.3.230&code=0161NRP&vmode=FULL.

PART 4: CONCLUSION

Boonstra, Evert, et al. "Neurotransmitters as Food Supplements: the Effects of GABA on Brain and Behavior." *Frontiers in Psychology*, Frontiers Media S.A., 6 Oct. 2015, www.ncbi.nlm.nih.gov/pmc/articles/PMC4594160/.

Breus, Michael. "Relaxation, a Strong Bio Clock, and Better Sleep: 5-HTP May Help." *Your Guide to Better Sleep*, 17 Apr. 2020, www.thesleepdoctor.com/2017/06/28/understanding-5-htp-relaxation-strong-bio-clock-better-sleep-5-htp-may-help/.

Brooks, Patricia L, and Peever, John H. "Unraveling the Mechanisms of REM Sleep Atonia." *Sleep*, Associated Professional Sleep Societies, LLC, Nov. 2008, www.ncbi.nlm.nih.gov/pmc/articles/PMC2579970/.

Camfield, David A, et al. "Acute Effects of Tea Constituents L-Theanine, Caffeine, and Epigallocatechin Gallate on Cognitive Function and Mood: a Systematic Review and Meta-Analysis." *Nutrition Reviews*, U.S. National Library of Medicine, Aug. 2014, www.ncbi.nlm.nih.gov/pubmed/24946991.

Cleveland Clinic "5 Surprising Facts About Sleep Apnea." *Health Essentials from Cleveland Clinic*, Health Essentials from Cleveland Clinic, 5 May 2020, health.clevelandclinic.org/5-surprising-facts-about-sleep-apnea/.

Foxe, John J, et al. "Assessing the Effects of Caffeine and Theanine on the Maintenance of Vigilance during a Sustained Attention Task." *Neuropharmacology*, U.S. National Library of Medicine, June 2012, www.ncbi.nlm.nih.gov/pubmed/22326943?dopt=Abstract.

Hasler, Gregor, et al. "Effect of Acute Psychological Stress on Prefrontal GABA Concentration Determined by Proton Magnetic Resonance Spectroscopy." *The American Journal of Psychiatry*, U.S. National Library of Medicine, Oct. 2010, www.ncbi.nlm.nih.gov/pubmed/20634372.

Hong, Ki-Bae, et al. "Sleep-Promoting Effects of the GABA/5-HTP Mixture in Vertebrate Models." *Behavioural Brain Research*, U.S. National Library of Medicine, 1 Sept. 2016, www.ncbi.nlm.nih.gov/pubmed/27150227.

Kimura, Kenta, et al. "L-Theanine Reduces Psychological and Physiological Stress Responses." *Biological Psychology*, U.S. National Library of Medicine, Jan. 2007, www.ncbi.nlm.nih.gov/pubmed/16930802.

Oksenberg A, Silverberg DS, Arons E, Radwan H. Positional vs non-positional obstructive sleep apnea patients: anthropomorphic, nocturnal polysomnographic, and multiple sleep latency test data. Chest. 1997 Sep;112(3):629-39.

Oksenberg A, Arons E, Greenberg-Dotan S, Nasser K, Radwan H. [The significance of body posture on breathing abnormalities during sleep: data analysis of 2077 obstructive sleep apnea patients]. [Article in Hebrew] Harefuah. 2009 May;148(5):304-9, 351, 350.

Mckeown. Patrick. "Buteyko Breathing Method For Snoring and Obstructive Sleep Apnea." *Buteyko Clinic*, buteykoclinic.com/sleepapnea/2019/

Portas, C M, et al. "Serotonin and the Sleep/Wake Cycle: Special Emphasis on Microdialysis Studies." *Progress in Neurobiology*, U.S. National Library of Medicine, Jan. 2000, www.ncbi.nlm.nih.gov/pubmed/10622375.

Portas, C M, et al. "Serotonin and the Sleep/Wake Cycle: Special Emphasis on Microdialysis Studies." *Progress in Neurobiology*, U.S. National Library of Medicine, Jan. 2000, www.ncbi.nlm.nih.gov/pubmed/10622375.

Stańska, Katarzyna, and Antonii Krzeski. "The Umami Taste: from Discovery to Clinical Use." *Otolaryngologia Polska* = *The Polish Otolaryngology*, U.S. National Library of Medicine, 30 June 2016, www.ncbi.nlm.nih.gov/pubmed/27387211.

Winkelman, John W, et al. "Reduced Brain GABA in Primary Insomnia: Preliminary Data from 4T Proton Magnetic Resonance Spectroscopy (1H-MRS)." *Sleep*, Associated Professional Sleep Societies, LLC, Nov. 2008, www.ncbi.nlm.nih.gov/pubmed/19014069.

Young, Simon N. "How to Increase Serotonin in the Human Brain without Drugs." *Journal of Psychiatry & Neuroscience : JPN*, Canadian Medical Association, Nov. 2007, www.ncbi.nlm.nih.gov/pmc/articles/PMC2077351/.

Young, Simon N. "How to Increase Serotonin in the Human Brain without Drugs." *Journal of Psychiatry & Neuroscience : JPN*, Canadian Medical Association, Nov. 2007, www.ncbi.nlm.nih.gov/pmc/articles/PMC2077351/.

Still confused what's keeping you up? Take the Sleep Quiz.

If you have trouble either getting to staying asleep, there is a good chance you have insomnia. Take the 2-minute sleep quiz to discover what could be causing you insomnia and determine what is keeping you from refreshing sleep.

To take the quiz visit:

SleepScienceAcademy.com/sleepquiz

About Devin Burke

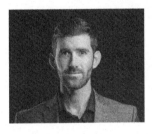
Devin Burke is an author, speaker and the chief energy office of Sleep Science Academy, a company specializing in helping exhausted insomniacs and high achievers get and stay asleep using a cutting edge unique holistic approach based in science.

He has inspired thousands of people through his books, videos, courses, coaching and keynotes.

For more information about Devin and Sleep Science Academy, please visit.

DevinBurke.com

About
Sleep Science Academy

We are on a mission to help the 40+ million people who suffer from insomnia to naturally get and stay asleep as soon as possible. Our proven system built by an expert and backed by science helps exhausted insomniacs who have "tried everything" and still can't sleep…sleep peacefully again in 8-weeks or sooner.

In our signature 8-week Insomnia Solved program, we help our clients eliminate sleep anxiety, reset their body's sleep system and leverage the world's most advanced sleep tracking technology to help them escape the "insomniacs paradox."

To learn more and see if you are a fit for what we offer go to:

SleepScienceAcademy.com

Acknowledgments

This book would not have been possible without the help and support of the following people:

My beautiful wife, Sonia - thank you for believing in me when I didn't believe in myself. Thank you for being my biggest fan and for all your love.

My incredible family; Mom, Dad, Dan, Brandon, Scott as well as the entire Burke, Iacovone and Richards family. I feel beyond blessed to have you all in my life.

My crew: You know who you are and I love you. Being connected to you all makes me better.

Amanda and Mom for editing.

Kirk for nailing the headshots.

All my past clients: You've taught me so much and for that I am grateful.

Last but certainly not least to all my mentors and teachers.

Did you enjoy this book?
Please don't forget to leave a review.

My mission is to get this book into the hands of the people who need it the most and your book review makes all the difference! Thank you so much for reading and reviewing.

To make this easy, you can visit

SleepAdvantageBook.com/review

Made in the USA
Monee, IL
25 April 2023

32420708R00083